Reader reviews

★ ★

A hea....

"Some poems made me smile or laugh out loud ... the brutal honesty and some made me cry (a lot) and there were many penny-dropping moments for me. I could relate to nearly all of them which was very scary.... that a total stranger could un-jumble my thoughts and feelings over the years and write them down in a book."

★★★★★

Honest, intelligent and beautiful

"The beauty of being autistic is in here along with the challenges of self-acceptance and self-compassion. I struggle with these things too and found this book very validating and - well, anything that makes you go a bit easier on yourself has to be a good thing."

★★★★★

The book that could be my autobiography

"It made me laugh and cry in equal measure as I recognised myself in your words."

★★★★★

"Reading this book was an act of compassion for myself. Poems were like a balm that soothed and aided digestion. Thank you for writing."

★★★★★

"Wow well… I relate to the authors words 100% which is hard to read but validating. Need more books like this, thank you."

★★★★★

Honest and relatable

"This is such a honest, open and helpful book. As a late-diagnosed neurodivergent person myself, I could really relate to the emotional rollercoaster in this book. The author has distilled a complex subject into an engaging and easy to understand format, breaking down some of the many aspects how neurodiversity presents in day to day life. I really loved the mixture of poems and personal experience. The fact it was told in real time as the writer comes to terms with her own feelings and challenges gave a real feeling of immediacy and allowed me as a reader to learn alongside her."

★★★★★

"An absolutely beautiful layout for a very important and impactful book - absolutely loved it"

★★★★★

Loved it

"Very relatable easy to read combination of poems and prose describing the experience of a late discovered autistic woman. Honest and raw."

MESS IS PROGRESS

A personal chronicle of an unmasking, late-diagnosed, Autistic woman

Hannah Walker

Foreword by
Flo Jones

Char, weirdos rule the world! Hannah x

Copyright © Hannah Walker 2024
Original Edition Published 2023
Revised Edition Published 2024
Foreword Copyright © Flo Jones 2024

All rights reserved.
Hannah Walker has asserted her moral right under the Copyright, Designs & Patent Act 1988 and no part of this work may be reproduced in any way without prior written consent of Hannah Walker.

ISBN 978-1-7385103-0-6

Cover design:
Hannah Walker
Cover fonts:
Personal Services by Daniel Hochard - imagex-fonts.com
Kingsman from Myfonts by Monotype

www.hannahpoems.co.uk
Facebook @hannahpoems
Instagram @hannah.poems

Foreword	5
About the Author	7
Introduction	8
How it began	9
The unmasking and healing process	10
An ode to... another bad night's sleep	13
Struggling thoughts	15
Call me crazy	17
Conversations in my head	20
Can we have some time	21
Really big font	22
Poem Fail	24
Decision making	25
Joy. Oops where did it go?	26
Wednesday Walks	27
You are brave	28
Dysregulation	29
A perfect excuse	30
"Unacceptable"	31
Being an Autistic mum	33
I Don't Remember	36
Glorious Natter	40
She's such a delight	41
Friendships IRL and online	42
Affirmations	46
Happy but sad, happy and sad	47
Time to leave the house	49
The call of the sea	50
Mondays suck	52

Spontaneous Bookshop	54
Wednesday of woe	55
Flexing my disability (or not as the case may be)	56
A green shiny	59
Sensory troubles	60
Mess is progress	61
Contemporary dance of the mind	**63**
Just say no	65
Success	66
Being Vulnerable	68
The trauma time capsule	69
Shopping – Sensory overwhelm	71
A little bit of a loner	72
Sensory seeking attention seeker	73
Rejection Prevention	75
RSD and me	**76**
It's ok to fucking age	79
Communication deficit	80
Breaking the cycle	81
A brave day	86
What would you say?	87
Showering	88
Monday Existential Crisis Day	90
Capacity Tuesday	91
Let down meltdown	93
Inaccessibility rant	**95**
Problem to be fixed	97
Fireworks	98
A Neurodivergent family	100
Never quite good enough	102

Befuddled Brain	104
The brain switch on	106
Why can't I cry?	108
Grief is not linear	**109**
A cautious burnout exit	111
A pledge	113
Dopamine delight	114
You are extraordinary	115
The ghost of my Christmases past	116
The car-crash of change	**117**
Trust my boundaries	121
Toxic validation seeker	122
Bang on brand	125
Where have all the safe foods gone?!	126
Rest & Remove	127
The pieces of me	128
You look nice	131
Dutch courage, social crutch	133
The misadventure of employment	**135**
Empathy Curse	142
Evangelical bralette pusher	144
The slug and pillow	145
Unmasking acceptance	146
Fight, flight and freeze	147
So flighty	148
Well shit, I'm disabled	149
A need to know basis	150
Finding her Autistic voice	151
100% Autistic	**152**
Burden	155

Local derby	156
The witches and the weirdos	157
Do not disturb	158
Bumps	159
We can learn a lot from a 6 year old	**160**
More goddamn forms	162
Failure	163
12 hours	164
Hair bobble	165
The closing of a year	167
Shedding the weight	169
Not my first rodeo	170
I am fierce	171
The can do and the cannots	172
Letter in my head	173
I'm sorry	174
The letter	**175**
For Mum & Dad	183
Four	184
Oh you're still here	185
Life is like a winter walk	186
Settle down now	187
Floordrobe	188
A walk on the beach	189
Overstimulated goblin	190
A body full of trauma	**191**
Two worlds collide	197
A kids bike	198
The tank is empty	199
Vermicelli noodles	200

Inner-child healing on wheels	201
Repeat after me	202
Weirdo magnet	**203**
Did we take over the world?	**204**
Love language	205
Purple buttons	206
Hello brain	**207**
Sugar-coated VA	210
Not a genie	211
Representation	212
Holy Sh**. Get out of my brain	**213**
Epilogue	**215**
Acknowledgements	**216**
Glossary of terms (Hannah's way)	**219**
Helpful resources	**224**

To my Neurodivergent friend
and your healing inner child:
you are enough
you are not too much
your emotions are valid
you are so worthy

To the future of our
glorious Autistic children:
may your struggles be less
as we fight for your
rights in society

We believe in you

Foreword

At first, I devoured this book
binged on it, like it was my comfort food
then once my appetite came back
I returned again to savour
all the words I'd left un-chewed

You meet one Autistic person
they say you've met one Autistic person
we're diverse, beautiful
and in a class of our own
and in truth that's how it felt at school
sat on squat and sweaty seats
doing group work on my own

That said and hear me out on this
there are strong threads
that tie us all together
in this case it felt more like a rope
so strong and steadfast was the link
between my own life
and the words I'd read
tales of despair, injustice
and at it's heart… hope

Perhaps I felt a fleeting discomfort
only due to the unsettling synchronicity
after a lifetime of feeling misunderstood
but now on paper was the friend
I'd sorely needed, the companion
I'd wanted to forge connection with
but never could

Once the book was read
my hunger was satisfied
I was soothed by waves
of comforting recognition
If your brain is wired differently
and you need sisterhood right now
I recommend you read
what Hannah has written

Flo Jones
participant on the documentary
Inside Our Autistic Minds

About the Author

Oh this is me... A photographer, mother and feminist living in the South West of England, spending as much time at the beach as possible. When I'm not beach side, I'll be cooking up a new project, probably for our little cottage and garden, both of which are in constant evolution. When I was young I always knew I would be doing something creative but my education was riddled with repercussions of being an undiagnosed Autistic & ADHD child. My reports consisted many a time of "she has so much potential, if only she could apply herself". Alas I fell into a variety of job roles none of which could go the distance. As I exited my twenties I went back to college and re-trained as a photographer, setting up my own business in 2012. Turns out there are a lot of us Neurodivergents in photography and finding my people was a pivotal part of discovering my true self.

I've been writing blogs for as long as I can remember, most around my special interests and often deeply personal. There was always a cloak of anonymity doing it online, although it was out in the world I didn't feel so exposed. In addition to my incognito online musings I have always been a fan of penning poems. For as far back as I can remember, there was the maudlin-emo pre-teen days of woe, to gifts of love for friends and this collection here is my public debut *shits pants* Ironic really, given the challenges I had studying GCSE English at school. How I hated those lessons but the contrast of how much I needed the written form to not only express but understand the constant monologue in my head.

Introduction

This chronicle began 2 months after I was diagnosed as Autistic and the subsequent utter burnout. My brain was so busy with so many things from the total trivial to the full-blown existential crisis that comes with being Neurodivergent and only just learning an absolutely crucial piece of my identity at 40 years old.

With three children spanning three decades, life was and always will be what I describe as organised chaos. My eldest was born when I was still so young at 17, followed by our first daughter in my twenties, then our youngest in my thirties. It has been a wild ride to say the least but they have all made me radiate with hope and pride, guiding me. Each one has taught me how to be a better human in their own unique ways.

Mess is Progress is built from chapters of writing during my unmasking revelations and the unfolding of my past with this new Autistic lens, and also poems - if you are new to poetry, you can think of them as extended relatable memes. The poems are catalogued in chronological order of which they were written - I wanted you to see the journey it took me on. There is also a Glossary of Terms at the end, written with explanations *my* way. There are many new words you may or may not have heard of before, since you started to explore Autism. Learn these and it will help you in your unmasking journey too.

How it began

In 2021 my daughter's teachers invited my husband and I in for a meeting - she was 15 years old at the time. We had been conversing with them for a while because something wasn't quite right with her learning and we couldn't work out what it was. We desperately wanted to support her and needed their help. That journey in itself hit a few bumps because we were initially met with a defensive response about their teaching methods. It wasn't until later when the Head of Year got involved and she broached us to suggest that our daughter may in fact be Autistic and asked us to begin the process for a referral and Autism Assessment.

We were pretty stunned by this, as it was not something we were expecting them to say. Sure she's always been pretty quirky but she was so damn smart and our own knowledge around Autism was limited to that of the general representation we see in media and of friends or family with Autistic boys. So of course once it had sunk in, I got straight into the research. Starting with the book *"Girls and Autism – Educational, Family and Personal Perspectives" by Barry Carpenter, Frances Happé and Jo Egerton* - My husband and I read it at the same time on our kindles, highlighting sections that related, I realised that I was highlighting for our daughter and what also rang true for me. Initially we thought, well it's going to have some similar things for me too because it's all we are reading and thinking about. By the time I finished that book I knew I had my whole life thus far staring right back at me. An onslaught of deep-diving research into Autistic girls and women ensued as I read more books, joined forums, read blogs, and followed Autistic content creators on Instagram. And yes, I completed every Autism questionnaire going. Hello new special interest.

Due to it nearly being time for our daughter to sit her GCSEs, her referral getting lost in the NHS ether for three months and starting again from the beginning, we made the decision to seek out a private practice for her assessment. I found a lovely local practice that followed all the NICE guidelines for assessment and it all snowballed from there. Initially, my entire focus was on her and getting her through a pretty long and gruelling (for an Autistic person with social anxiety!) process. I made a note in my brain that once this process was done, I can allow myself to seek my own assessment. Erin was diagnosed as Autistic in March 2022 and a month later I began the process again, for me this time. I appreciate I was in a privileged position to be able to go private and although I had already reached my own conclusion that I too was Autistic, I couldn't shake the need for a formal diagnosis from my brain - I needed validation, I needed to understand more and I needed to stop feeling like an imposter.

The unmasking and healing process

What I wasn't prepared for was the grief and confusion and constant processing that stems from an official diagnosis, which I received in July 2022 after many sessions, lots of emails (because I would always remember more after a session!) and a corroboration interview with my husband.

I had started seeing a therapist back in 2021 (again) because I was unpacking a lot of things around it all but she openly admitted she didn't know an awful lot about autism in girls and women. So I made the decision to seek out one that did (and I urge anyone going through the same to find a Neuro-affirming therapist). This meant my therapy was going online because living in the outer sticks of the South West countryside there aren't many around! I was quite dubious initially about doing weekly therapy in front of my computer, but it was better than I expected. I had already started an attempt to journal with my busy brain, then my therapist during one of our earlier sessions, suggested I make an effort to write for as many pages as I could each day. I had used poetry as a child to write my feelings down before and as an adult have written many poems for friends, family, and special occasions. Suddenly this journaling turned into poetry too and before I knew it I was writing a couple of poems a day.

As an Autistic woman, understanding, processing and verbalising my feelings is a gargantuan task but the freedom I found with my own written word was this new way to communicate. Sometimes I started a therapy session with one of my poems, to begin the conversation of how my week had been. This communication wasn't solely an outward tool, internally I was communicating to myself. I was sorting and sifting through my brain and feelings and unmasking for the first time. Most importantly I was unmasking to myself through my own written words.

It's been a powerful tool and with some encouragement (thank you Zena) I decided it could possibly help other people in my position too and so here it is. My post-diagnosis, poetic memoir with a smattering of rambles, from yours truly.

An ode to... another bad night's sleep

Slowly stirring
laying on the sofa
silk eye mask
earplugs in
belly bubbling
morning IBS

Thud, thud, thud
in my ears, woosh
as my blood pumps
a song going
around and around
my brain

What even is
that song?
with the woosh
and the bubbles
and the song

The words
object permanence
begin to
rattle and bounce
again and again
what does it
mean again?

Woosh
bubble
song
"object permanence"

I begin to count
2 hours plus 3 hours
I definitely need
more sleep

Woosh
thud thud
"object permanence"

I think I dreamt
of holidays
between the overthinking

It's Harry bloody Styles!
god my brain
please be quiet
and you bubble belly

Object fucking permanence

I can feel my teeth
game-over now
as I roll off the sofa
wobbly and blinking

Bathroom
brush teeth

Struggling thoughts

Struggling thoughts,
what does it mean
to struggle?

I'm exhausted
everything seems
too much
am I too much?

Why are tasks
so hard
to even think
let alone do

As I start a
list in my head
the overwhelm
absorbs me

The layers
of trauma
enter my brain

Layer upon layer
deaths, changes
and challenges

Coping but not
the minute tasks
become mountains

Hygiene and chores
impossible chasms

how? just how?
not now,
I can't.

The bare minimum
to survive
as I feel like
an empty shell

Robotic almost
but much less
efficient.

Call me crazy

When the burnout hits
the spiral starts
existential crisis time
back again
worries about how
others will perceive me
and a long life
of not knowing
or understanding
my whole story

It is all internalised
don't act crazy
don't let them see
show them who
they expect you to be
but when it's all held in
it makes the spiral deeper

So now with the knowledge
where do I go?
what do I show?
I have names and reasons
for what is happening
but I still hesitate
the fear of rejection
ever prevalent

Burnout, shutdown, meltdown
sounds like excuses
for what I really am
what I've been called
my whole life:

hard work
uncooperative
lazy
emotional
hysterical
dramatic
moody
irrational
disobedient
needy
unorganised
erratic

So many words
and none are right
I'm Autistic
the one word
that makes it all make sense
the social exhaustion
the sounds and the noises
the struggles for years
of not letting the crazy show

So what do I need?
love, patience and understanding
time to grieve
time to heal
cuddles and quiet time
soft blankets and low light
and my age-old friend
VALIDATION

But to receive this
I need to let it out
how do I get passed

my force field
of self preservation?
it's a scary and
vulnerable place
that my exceptional
masking has protected
me from for so long.

But I am tired once more
burnout is back
I can manage this better
now that I know I'm Autistic
that simple life hack
though it seems so foreign

Ask. For. Help.

Conversations in my head

Practiced and constructed
conversations in my head
every detail I want you to know
I mull it over, think it out
my feelings portrayed
and my thoughts explained
it seems so easy in my brain
rehearsed and planned
conversations in my head
a busy mind yet the words
are always left unsaid.

this poem was brought to you
by another fucking sleepless night
3am, wish me luck!

Can we have some time

Can we have some time please
just some to process
who am I now?
I really have never known me.

Can we have some time please
time to rest from trauma
to unfold these feelings
to let them out and let me be.

Can we have some time please
a safe space to really talk
to move forward the right way
and to finally meet my needs.

Can we have some time please
no work, no chores
just cuddles indoors
some quiet time with no TV

Can we have some time please
to wander in the wildlife
to chat, hold hands
and to feel that autumn breeze.

Can we have some time please
to smile and laugh all day
to play games on the floor
to listen to the call of the sea.

Really big font

I interrupt this poem broadcast with a ramble of thoughts that couldn't possibly be put into a few choice words. When I first read through my assessment report and diagnosis I cried. So much crying, snot tears, the lot. It's no wonder post diagnosis is a time of grief and my god the processing that goes on. I didn't just read it once either, glutton for punishment this one. Also there is the constant imposter syndrome, despite having it all there in black and white, intimate details about my entire life with deficit upon deficit of everything I am unable to do or struggle with because I am Autistic.

It seems when it's my daughter having her report I could give her the pep talk of, "hey sweetheart, these assessments are done on deficits alone and none of your amazing qualities are listed so don't be too disheartened by it. It's also more about being in a society that isn't set up for you, rather than you not being good enough for society". Yeah I preached it... I did not however, practice it.

I was properly grief stricken. I felt physically wounded by it. My heart ached so hard for younger me and all she had endured. Some would argue that she turned out ok in the end, look how strong you are etc, but I didn't feel strong - I felt lost all the time but carried on regardless.

Then the intrusive thoughts began, especially as I read over my husband's part of the report (repeatedly whilst crying). Why was he still with me? What did he ever see in me? You name it, I thought it. One afternoon, sat out in the garden after going through the conversation in my head for a number of days, I finally, somehow, expelled the words from my mouth.

The regret started to bubble up immediately, as I am so used to keeping these deeply personal and often unsubstantiated thoughts to myself. My heart was in my throat, I felt sick, am I actually going to be sick? Maybe. Oh god I'm sweating, it's hot isn't it?! Crap what have I done this for?

Of course there's a reason I married this man, although not one for talking too openly about emotions he managed to diffuse this bomb in my head in one swooping response of light-hearted humour. First he reminded me that I haven't changed because I have a diagnosis, I'm still the exact same person he fell in love with. Ok, valid point, but maybe you could just write up my good points, an antidote if you will. To which he responded, "I can but I'd have to use a single page and a really big font".

Poem Fail

I tried to write a poem today
but it was a bit shit
so I ripped it out and ripped it up
and now it no longer exists.

I guess I am a bit distracted
with the weekend plans
packing the car
oh look a message
oh shit I need to write a list
oh shit I should give the kitchen man
the sink and handles
fuck I need to get fuel
oh for f-sake
I still haven't eaten breakfast
mustn't forget the shampoo.

I tried to write a poem today
but it was a bit shit.
so I ripped it out
and now I guess this is it.

Decision making

Decision making
can I get an "ugh"
so brain taxing

Why are there
so many choices
questions a plenty
an abundance of voices

What to wear
what's for dinner
shall we do this
shall we do that

I need time
for my brain to process
which rarely happens
and frankly why
it all fells like
a big fucking mess

Joy. Oops where did it go?

There are so many things that
bring me ultimate joy.

It sucks when I'm burned out
I'm like a sad broken toy.

I love autumn walks
in the crisp fresh air
blue skies, orange leaves
the wind in my hair.

But instead I'm at home
so very tired, but trying
school runs, phone calls, emails
adulting sort of and inside I'm dying…

I'm dying to re-ignite that spark
to spend time on my interests
but instead I'm just sat in the dark

I wish I knew how long
this burnout will last
so I can get back to my joy
and move on from my past.

Wednesday Walks

A much needed walk outside
talking nonsense with a good friend
tractors, orchards, sunshine and clouds
sheep grazing among the apple trees
not entirely sure on the route

A mob of mooing cows
beautiful green ferns lining the way
trees uprooted and on their side
some so old even their roots
look like actual trees themselves

A delicious brunch before
the stomp back begins
sugar high laughter as we
share daft stories

I bloody love autumn
and our Wednesday walks.

You are brave

"I'm scared" she says
as I hold her hand
it's ok to be scared
remember you are brave
you can do this,
to be brave
is to be scared
but do the thing anyway.

"I'm scared" she says
"But I really want to do it"
I believe you can sweetheart
I'm here and I will watch you.
you don't know this
but I'm scared for you too.

You are brave
and you did it.
you were so proud.
I clapped and
I cheered and
held back the tears.

You were scared
and you were brave.
I'm so proud of you.

Miss Mila moon, your first cross country race
age 6yrs & 8months, with 110 other girls
in your group… wow!

Dysregulation

Things that help me regulate after dysregulation and/or a big fat burnout.

Quiet time
cosy time
time wrapped in a blanket
comfy clothes

Familiar programmes
especially when I can release a big ole cry.
favourite playlist
simple food

Standing in the garden
turned towards the warm sunshine
playing with my hair

Writing in my notebook
the sound of the sea
and if I am able then a dip is pretty good too.

A perfect excuse

Today is a wait around day
the worktop man's measure day
the sky engineer installs a new box day.

It's a rainy day
a perfect excuse day
to take some time day

A quick tidy up day
leave them to their work day
casually practice some French day

Got a wedding tomorrow prep day
eat super noodles in bed day
get excited about interiors day

Looking forward to the weekend day
beanie hat and big cardigan day.

Let's get a takeaway day and
light the log burner day

Happy Friday kinda day.

"Unacceptable"

The system is fucked
why is it all a fight?
to be Neurodivergent
in a society
that does not accommodate
who you are
means you are in
a constant battle
we are the advocates
of our daughter's future
but when people
the very authority
that should want
the best for your child
and their education
take your requests
for accommodations
for support
to help us as parents
help them
as a slight on their ability
a black mark
to their name
like we are the ones
not playing the right game
to be offended
by our need
to meet her needs
and to call us
in our quest
"Unacceptable"
why should it feel
like an us against them

but no matter
your defence
your crap reaction
or lack of support
we have won
this small fight
and we will win them
again and again
because the system
is fucked
and society
is not made for us
but with every
Neurodivergent
we fight the fight
and we make
the world better
with all our Autistic,
unwavering might!

This poetic rant was brought to you for the fight we've endured for our Autistic teenager during her GCSEs.

Being an Autistic mum

We're just talking about Autistic motherhood here as this is the only perspective I know and have the experience to share about. I'm sure this can be similar to that of dads or non-binary parents too.

Parenting is hard, full stop. No matter your neurological brain setup, raising well-rounded humans without mistakes is impossible and there will always be challenges along the way. The thing that gets me, being an Autistic mum and raising Autistic children is the constant fight we have to endure. I am forever armed for battle. It's exhausting.

The problem is the lack of knowledge, understanding, training and support in our education system. The information is out there and my god it's frustrating because I feel pretty clued up on it all now (hello hyper fixation) and sometimes I forget that most school staff do not know what I now do, and it is their actual job to recognise the signs. What's even more frustrating is that it didn't take me that long to discover this information. We have so much at our fingertips, I kind of feel like there really is no excuse to be so ill-educated about something that affects so many students.

When I was a child, it was all about the naughty little boys having ADHD or the non-verbal Autistic boys that got additional support. You were naughty and disciplined, called manipulative (for having needs), sometimes just a lost cause. When my dad was a child, he was constantly getting the cane (pretty certain he is Autistic and ADHD) - he once described his younger self as a lost wretch which made me sadder than you can believe because he was consistently let down by those that should have nurtured him. But it's 2022 now and what is our excuse for still persistently failing Neurodivergent children in our schools and throughout society?

It is literally a full time job being on top of the school providing the right support, filling out forms and going to appointments for Neurodivergent children. Throw into the mix that I too am Autistic and ADHD and wow, what a cocktail of headfuckery. I have an immense injustice warrior trait and I will die on this hill of stepping up and raging this war for my children, because they deserve it and well, I never had it. I will fight until I take my last breath for them and whilst I am here fighting, I am also nurturing my own inner child and that shit hits home hard.

The complicated place it leaves me at times, burned out to the max but carrying on regardless with the weight of the world on my shoulders, in turn raises my sensory processing issues, sleep deprivation (because my brain doesn't stop) and some days I just cannot function. Therapy has helped me to realise that I do need rest and should take it because then I can be more functional after some down time. I urge you to do this too because it is all a lot. Remembering to do things that bring me joy is so important and sharing that pure joy with my kids too. It doesn't even have to be much - a kitchen disco of uninhibited dancing to the beat is a firm favourite for all of us.

The amount of times I've wanted to just stick two fingers up at the capitalist society we live in as it destroys our souls. Let's start a commune in the woods by a lake and share skills, lighten the load of life for each other and celebrate each other's individuality. We can teach our children about this incredible planet we inhabit and embrace each other's interests and happiness because that far outweighs creating submissive, mechanical workers lining the pockets of the rich.

swishes skirt barefoot in the daisies whilst foraging berries and firewood with the kids - we all jump into the lake for a wild swim as the sun sets

If only it was that easy!

I Don't Remember

I don't remember
I don't remember much
of my childhood
there are very few
things that stick
in my mind

I remember roller skating
and playing dogs
I remember fishing for newts
and watching hedgehogs at dusk.

I don't remember much
about school
I remember finding it
so very confusing
the majority of the time

I remember falling
asleep in assembly
I remember being nervous
about standing up front
for the birthday song

I remember having
a complete meltdown
because the first
school photos I ever had
I opened it
you open it you buy it
I did not know.
I would be in so much trouble
I was so distraught that

my friend's mum
bought the photo.

I remember the smell
of the crayons
during wet play.
I remember pissing my pants
a lot.

I remember giving
a dead fluffy bumble bee
a burial on a super hot day.

I remember the kid
who literally ate the pencils.

Up to junior school
I remember very vaguely
our old school building

I remember the walk
to school more than
the day there.
especially that one time
it snowed and
my neighbour was walking
back the wrong way
it was closed!

I remember angry teachers
I remember the best
bit about swimming
was afterwards when
we got to look at books
on the grass whilst

waiting for everyone.
I remember the worst bit
was not feeling like
I could do it
that I was actually
going to drown
and Mr R
just being angry
when I asked for help.

I remember when
they built the new school
I didn't like the change.

It was right next
to the senior school
and the boys would
ask questions
I didn't understand
through the fence
that separated
our two schools
like "are you a virgin"

I don't remember
the lessons much
I remember Mr A
picked on the new girl
so I made friends with her

I remember Mr E
spat when he talked
so I avoided
being in the line of fire.

I remember never
really fitting in
or having someone
to play with at break.
until the new boy started
and we became friends
we watched hedgehogs together

I remember I loved
him a lot and
how distraught
I was when
he moved away.

I remember wanting
spikey hair
and another older
child calling me
a brother to my sister

Turns out I remember
a fair bit after all
and I haven't even
started on senior school.

Glorious Natter

I wrote the date and
had a subject in mind
however my sister called
and we spent over an hour
just chatting on FaceTime

Now my mind has
gone blank
however my heart
is full and warm.

So that is a great thing
because it's much less busy
in the ole grey matter
it's amazing how a call
with the right person
at the right time
can make all the difference
thank you Gemma for
our glorious natter

She's such a delight

Before I knew my Autistic identity
I used to believe that I was
suffering frequent mental breakdowns
I mostly hid these from everyone.
I shared a made up reality
one of a super fun and outgoing
kind of person.
oh the confidence she had,
what a beacon of light.
I mean the drugs and alcohol helped
she made friends, held conversations
danced and joked, what a delight.
what they didn't see
were the regular meltdowns
the anxiety, the fear
and the shutdowns.
the sobbing to sleep feeling so lonely
despite being surrounded by friends
my secrets locked up, my true self hidden
who are these people, they don't even know me.

Friendships IRL and online

It may be obvious by now that when you're Autistic, especially undiagnosed, you spend a lot of time feeling like you don't really have any proper close friends. Even when you have friends. Sometimes you have friends of convenience, you and they are at the same time and place of life but when you split onto different paths you never see them again or don't even think about them (and I'm sorry to those people if you're reading this, but look up object permanence, Autistics do this with people too). They are quite literally out of sight and out of mind.

I distinctly remember finding it so utterly bizarre that my husband's friendship group, when I met him at 28 years old, were the group of boys he went to school with. Baffling. I had no friends left from school. I had a few friendship infatuations when I was young and was left inconsolable when those friendships broke down, which ultimately they always did. The jealousy I felt when I looked at my peers who seemed to be able to hang onto their bezzies, what was wrong with me, why couldn't I do it?

Thankfully by 18 years old I had discovered the clubbing scene, house music and the veritable pit of dopamine that was dancing (stimming) my ass off in a room full of strangers where I didn't have to talk to people if I didn't want to *sorry what was that, I can't hear you over the music*. Eyes closed feeling the bass and waving my arms in the air. Unless of course you are in the chill out room where you do converse with complete no-ones about utter bullshit yet none of the small talk. Or better still the ladies toilets where apparently you can just go for a box-room full of your own hype team of absolute strangers. If you're ever having a down day, I urge you to get wasted and hang out in the ladies toilets. The compliments and camaraderie in those places are second to none.

I will never forget the day I met what I would say is my first (and still outstanding) best friend Pickle. One night in a club after we had the best time dancing, she just wrapped her arms around me and shouted "I think you're brilliant" and I genuinely couldn't believe that someone I barely knew had come to this conclusion about me? Brilliant. This was the beginning of me realising there were people out there for me and over the different eras of my life, I began collecting them like rare treasures and holding onto them as well as I could through the transitions of growing up. My adult birthday parties felt like a celebration of said collection, where I would get them all together and the only thing connecting them was me and they were my treasures. There would be the odd colleague, someone I met a house party, a neighbour, even would you believe it, mum friends. Also I highly recommend dropping off a Krispy Kreme donut to try and make friends when pregnant. This is what Emily did as the other preggo in the village. What an icebreaker! I opened my front door to a Biscoff delight being held out to me by this cool mum from the school with a matching baby belly to mine. Needless to say she was scooped up into my friend treasure box with the rest of the best. If anyone were to ever print out our messenger conversations I think it would be like unravelling intestines, it would just go on and on and would definitely contain a lot of shit (as well as an inexplicable amount of memes and GIFs).

If we're still friends and our lives have changed, evolved, moved, grown, then congratulations, you're in the box too. Even if we don't talk as often as we'd like to, if we are still in touch (no matter how sporadically) it's because you are wonderful.

Despite often forgetting I'm probably considered old now at forty, I do have to remind myself that I existed before social media and the world being accessible through your phone. Around 2004, I discovered online forums and wow, this is much easier than chatting in real life. Conversing about things that mattered intimately and deeply to me was always such a challenge with friends and family, I internalised so much. My first dabble in forums when I was trying to get pregnant was a revelation. I obsessively got involved, these women were all trying to do the same thing as me and we could anonymously support each other, propping up our laptops on the sofa (no iPhones then!) and chatting. It became a special interest of which I whole-heartedly threw myself into. I was a moderator, I read up and researched everything to get pregnant and later after succeeding, joined a "Birth Board" where we were all due in the same month. I wrote my own blog and wrote for Babycentre's blog. I was balls deep in this online life. As the internet got more accessible it got even deeper, the advent of social media like Facebook allowed me to connect and continue relationships easier. I am still in touch now 17 years later with some of those women. Do you remember when everyone first got Facebook? There were people coming out of the woodwork I hadn't thought about for years or even remembered that we were friends. One person sent me a private message saying how gutted she was when I dropped out of college and abandoned her. I hand on heart didn't even remember she was there let alone that we were close. But then again I found college to be one big trauma to my senses, hence the quitting, so that's probably another thing my brain has protected me from remembering too much of.

This is a habit that has continued over the years for each and every special interest - find an online community for it. So naturally when I became a photographer, I did the same and now have some of the best photographer friends IRL as well as online, bloody loads of us are Autistic or ADHD too. More treasures for the box. I did the same with Volkswagens when we bought our first camper-van, stand up paddle boarding, genealogy and writing and author groups. Last but no means least, I am finally finding some Autistic spaces too.

Online socialising isn't without its drama though. Countless times I was called rude, blunt or intimidating for simply answering a question honestly. I didn't know I was Autistic at the time but I've had much abuse from people who didn't get my direct nature. Apparently you're supposed to lie or heavily sugar-coat responses to Neurotypicals - who knew?!

Affirmations

Not everyone has to like me
I don't need their validation to be happy

I don't need to go to all
the social events to prove
I am likeable

Content is home

Money isn't important
in being successful because
burnout is brutal

Meeting my needs isn't selfish
it's a necessity
of survival.

Happy but sad, happy <u>and</u> sad

It is possible to be happy
in your relationship
with your home and
your being
AND to be in a state
of grief, of processing
so much to unpack
your brain is like
a spaghetti junction
at rush hour
throwing up memories
with the new lens
of "I am Autistic"

And it is painful
to see those memories
in this new light
the countless times
you've been let down
by those who should
have nurtured and
supported you.
how you learnt
to shut everything up
inside yourself
to protect yourself

It is ok to be
in love and loved
and to still need
this time to go back
to help you understand
how to move forward

and to grow
it's bloody exhausting though.

Time to leave the house

Understanding and
working out when,
when you actually
need to go out of the house
and not when you think
you are just missing out.

Like tonight, I needed
to leave the house
after weeks of hermit-ness
and it wasn't that I felt
I had to be sociable
it's because I genuinely
needed a change of scenery.

And it felt good
and we bumped into friends
and we chatted about life
and parenting and politics
and nothing was forced
or weird
and it was just what I needed.

And the moon was so bright
on the walk home.
it was time well spent
and I socialised on my terms

Bravo to me!

The call of the sea

There's space on the beach
and the sun is like glitter
dancing on the sea

Dulcet tones of an
acoustic busker
muffled sounds of people
but no overwhelming crowds
the sun has a gentle warmth
across the surface of my skin

As I slip silently out of my clothes
and pad gently across the sand
holding onto your little hand
and our toes reach the shore
it is cold but comforting

Ankle deep now and giggling
through the surprise
of the temperature
we smile at each other
as the sea liberates us

enveloped by rollers
the chill biting at our limbs
cheekily nipping as we submit
to the call of the sea

swimming stretching and playing
in the big beautiful blue
movement for warmth

Your teeth sing a chatter
as we head back to the sand
for dry clothes

The ocean has cleansed
us of worries and
left joy in it's place.

Mondays suck

It's Monday
apparently World Mental Health Day
which for me is ironic
as I think Mondays are my lowest
I'm recognising a pattern
of the ebbs and flows
and Mondays suck
not because I have to get up
and drive to work
joys of being my own boss
but I guess it's the change
from the weekend
with more time and more joy
it's like I wake up with a loss
back to the monotony
alarm clocks, school runs
chores and yes probably
at least *some* work
but now I have spotted
the pattern
I'm learning
to go easy on myself
on Mondays, along with
season changes
return to term time
post school holidays
shorter days and
colder nights
they can all frankly
get in the bin

See also: recipe changes to favourite foods, shops no longer stocking the eyeliner you've always used, last minute plan changes, being late for anything. Get in the bin.

Spontaneous Bookshop

I walked into a little bookshop today
I've passed it so many times
admiring the books in the window.
for some reason today
I had the urge to actually enter
I'm so glad I did
because it was wonderful.

A carefully curated store of delight
books I've not seen or even heard of
standing tall, meticulously placed
beautiful book covers
art pieces in their own right
with tantalising titles and tales.

I wanted to buy so many
and curl up in a cosy chair
in a shard of Autumn sunlight
I'd read and read
and then read some more.

When that book is finished
I could deliberate over the next
striking cover and elaborate description
that enticed my brain into buying
ready for me to explore.

The joy they would bring lined on a shelf
talent in words and pictures.
somehow I managed to hold back
and bought just the one so I can repeat
this sublime, spontaneous encounter
and return to the bookshop for more.

Wednesday of woe

Wednesday of woe!
I am unwell,
physically ill.
my throat is raw
and tonsil is raging
I've had a fitful day
dosing off
reading a bit
painkillers around the clock

It's frustrating to think
oh I need a sick day
to rest my weary body.
guilt free naps
and help with the kids.

Why is it easier to
take the time out
and to even ask for help
when the pain is
obviously physical?

Flexing my disability (or not as the case may be)

I have had a few days off
from writing because
well I've been quite poorly
navigating an illness
and being Neurodivergent
is a wild ride!

I actually had my
tonsils removed when
I was twenty one.
they were ravaged
they were gnarly
and I almost died
after contracting a quinsy
whilst in an abusive relationship

So here I am
almost twenty years later
throat swelling
no sleep
and a large portion
of PTSD on the side.
3am I awake the husband
I need to go to A&E

Somehow amidst my panic
I picked up a book
my notebook and pens
earplugs and eye mask
a revelatory moment
of Autistic clarity

At the reception desk
I was told I had to
go in alone
(fucking Covid, again!)
my mind was screaming:
"but you're Autistic
tell them you need him"

Alas I did not
because I am not yet
able to flex my disability
when in need of help,
conversations with friends,
sure, open and chatty
when I need help?
that'll be a nope then

So I go in alone
after a tearful hug goodbye
and to my surprise
I'm seen quite soon.
I am given liquid morphine
though it didn't help much
and something else
in an oral liquid
to reduce the swelling

Blood test, IV fluids
bruised arms, throat spray,
observations.
then one more blood test
and I'm sent back to
the bright and noisy
waiting room

So very bright!
earplugs in, eye mask on.
feeling very pleased
with earlier me
packing my bag
in a panic
but still mindfully

I'm finally called back
by the doctor.
who talks me through
the prescription,
tablets – my nemesis.
I plead for liquid,
he assumes because
of my throat

I tell him I always
have liquid medicine
unless it's a very specific
small, sugar-coated tablet.
he asks me have I always
been like this?

Yes, yes I have
but I still don't say
I'm Autistic
and it's always been
a huge sensory issue

So I thank the kind man
take the prescription.
Thanks.

A green shiny

Having butchered my skin
on my fingers
nibbling with my teeth
I purchased my first
my very own
fidget toy
it's green (my favourite)
and shiny
very shiny
and it is twisty
and so unbelievably
satisfying.

Sensory troubles

Sensory things that have
troubled me today;

The smell of my sick husband
in the morning.

My god, do not breathe
near me

The constant feeling of a hair
on my face

The throb of the skin on
my right thumb of my own
causing with my teeth

My feet being too hot
my feet being too cold

The husband's sick sounds,
coughing and sniffing

The bubbles in the bath
making too much noise

The dripping of rain water
not the good sort, the missing gutter kind.

The cat smelling of horses

Mess is progress

As I shuffle through
the spilled contents of my brain
it's too much again.
there's so much to remember
so much to even process
my life as I look back,
childhood, relationships
the here and now,
parenting, adulting, renovating
mess is progress

To have the beautiful home
we first tear down some walls
dig some holes, tip out the old
the mess is progress

Accepting, unmasking
and understanding
mess is progress

Unlearning the masked behaviours
is realising the damage they've caused,
people pleasing, rejection sensitive,
mirroring, trying so hard to fit in
mess is progress

A lifetime of fawning
meeting everyone else's needs
or die trying
the mess, so much mess

The revelation that
my needs too can be met
Bless this mess and
all it's progress

Contemporary dance of the mind

Sometimes when I look back through what I've written, it doesn't surprise me the misdiagnosis rate of Autistic women and girls. The back and forth of my emotions and my being. The up and down of the good and the bad days. The hyper-motivated days and the "can't move from the same position" days. It is a beautiful mess and so worth it all, even those days that are tough because there is so much healing taking place.

I have a very visual brain, I can remember things by sight in my mind like a photograph or a video and can create images in my minds-eye very easily (albeit mashed together from past visuals my brain has collected). I have a filing system that I can see myself pulling things out of (it's not organised but it's there). Pain can be seen in my head and felt in my heart.

When I read back I can see a lone contemporary dancer emotively dancing out the journey I'm going on. She is delicate yet strong, rolls, spins and twists with grace across the floor. You know she is feeling each beat and moment in time as she goes. Sometimes it feels like she steps back but she is always eventually propelling forward to a place of acceptance and peace. There will be a breath-taking crescendo as the piece comes to a gentle end that leaves us both overcome, tears silently cascading down our faces as we reach the point of finally knowing who we are.

It's a damn shame I can't actually dance like her in my head because I think that would be incredible. The point of this dance in my mind is to say, this isn't a simple route from A to B and I'm getting that now. It takes time and perseverance but I am so bloody willing to put the effort in.

Working on boundaries and digging deep to discover my core values after a lifetime of masking is where the magic happens. It's where I'm going anyway!

Just say no

Declining an invitation
after 40 years of
learning the societal expectation
I always believed you had
to provide a suitable reason

However with my concoction
of RSD, autism and anxiety
my need to please meant
I would over divulge
and provide a full and
intricately detailed explanation

I tried a new thing today
and simply said I wouldn't
be able to make it
and hope they have a splendid shindig

Shortly followed by some
intense and unnecessary overthinking
because the inviter was fine!
nobody died

Success

What is success?
I have been taught
to be successful is
to achieve status
within my career
of climbing a hierarchy
that I never
really bought into

For me to achieve this,
is to successfully ruin myself
chasing after a belief
that is not my own
pushing past the pain
to get there
with something to prove
to family to strangers
a perilous path for
my wellbeing

I want to successfully
love myself for
who I am
to educate my mind
that I am worthy of love
and to represent
this love
this value
and this worth
as success to my children

Because they are worthy
of it all

no matter what they
grow up to be or who
is fortunate to be loved by them

Being Vulnerable

Being vulnerable
is scary.
Not knowing how
someone will react
is scary.

Cracking my shield
open for you to see
is vulnerable
and scary.

But I understand
to connect
is to communicate.
Some discomfort
and fear will
hopefully be
replaced with
belonging and safety.

The trauma time capsule

There is a box
inside my brain
that has been
filled up and locked up

like a time capsule
buried with memories.

Except this is
full of trauma
big and small

shut up
dug down deep
and never to
be shared at all.

There has been
an unexpected
excavation

it dinged the lid
and ripped it open

and now these
files so neatly
packed away,

are tumbling out
in a tornado
each one appearing
at any random time
on any random day.

So like a reader
at the end of
a news show.

I'm shuffling them
trying to organise
the thoughts

but really have
no idea where they go.

Shopping - Sensory overwhelm

Just an hour
one simple tock
around the clock
my senses assaulted
so much shiny
loads of texture
Halloween
Christmas
Kitchen
Bedroom
Candles
so many candles
different aromas
mostly offensive
a few pleasant
just one hour
in the shop
climb into the car
it's 10:30am
and I am wiped out
well hello
sensory overwhelm.

A little bit of a loner

A little bit of a loner
that's how you described
my wonderful daughter.
but it's ok because
she is a good and kind girl
who works hard and
plays by the rules,
a joy to teach.

Except we know she
isn't particularly happy
and at just 6 years old
she has anxiety.
but to you she's doing well
in her subjects,
like that is most important.
when she is clearly
struggling so much socially.

She has a thirst
for knowledge but
a need for meaningful
friendships and connection too.
She is an incredible child
but until you can see
past her academics,
deep thoughtfulness
and vast vocabulary.
will you ever be able
to meet her needs?

We need to help her thrive
and I need the school on my side.

Sensory seeking attention seeker

Brush my hair
but not the same place
over and over.

The sensory sweet spot
is underneath
from the nape of my neck
and the back of my ears.

Stroke my back
but not in small bits
or aforementioned sin
of the same spot.

Hug me tight,
fully wrapped
and long enough
for the tension release.

Cover me with a blanket
and fluffy socks.

If I'm having some
time out, check in,
so that I know you care.

A hot drink
a fizzy drink
lighting a fire but
also opening a window.

Let's go watch a sunset

or listen to the sea
a wild swim
live music.

Each of these
are flipping glorious to me

Rejection Prevention

Sometimes I think
you hate me
and the thought
burrows into my being
I plummet into sadness
then into protection and anger
and begin to try and
distance from you
to cushion the blow
of when you admit it
and leave me.

RSD and me

RSD – Rejection Sensitivity Dysphoria, three words that when I first discovered them, my mind was blown. The countless times and years I have been in such physical pain from rejection or even just perceived rejection is too vast to quantify. It's really hard to describe exactly how it feels but I thought I would at least try.

It's like a simultaneous shield punch in the gut from Lagertha Lothbrok whilst your heart is being shredded to tiny pieces by Villanelle. The grand finale feels like Eleven, of Stranger Things, mind-melt-throwing you across the room á la Henry and sending you through the gate to the Upside Down. It's no wonder that RSD can result in many, many panic attacks, right?

I believe that RSD is linked with both ADHD and Autism, and I'm certain I am both. It is hard for me to understand people's intentions, read between the lines and such like. I would often misread a situation, get a tone or action wrong and catapult myself full pelt into the outer reaches of the RSD stratosphere. I remember the troubles this caused in relationships, if he didn't say "I love you" back quick enough, a small snarky comment, a nonplussed response to something I was excited about or simply just being too busy to reply to me about something so insignificant it shouldn't have actually mattered. The pain and subsequent overthinking began. Not reserved only for partners but also friends, family, teachers, colleagues. It makes life really fucking confusing, and agonising. Autistic me would resort to going non-verbal for safety, sometimes a panic attack or meltdown would come first, my flight response (which has always been a favourite for my survival mode) would also kick in, off she goes!

The absolute worst memory I have of my Autistic, RSD mash-up would be when I was 16 and pregnant. Unsurprisingly my relationship had broken down and although we had remained friends, I was bereft thinking I would now be alone forever. At a friends 18th birthday party, I happened to see him leave with another girl. I had no hard cold facts and we weren't together anymore but the aforementioned physical pains began to my gut, heart and entire body. At first I ran (waddled maybe). I found a quiet step on a dark street on my own and just sat and tried to ride out the panic attack. A friend found me and took me home after not being able to get any response from me, as I was non-verbal. My mum was obviously really concerned; her pregnant teenage daughter had gone mute, as tears rolled down her face, sat, stock still on her bed. She did what she thought was best and took me to A&E. I still could not speak - I was asked if I'd taken any drugs (I looked that bad, and no I had not) but I could not use my voice. As the event got more and more traumatic, the less I had the ability to just say what was wrong. Blood tests ensued and my RSD further spiralled as in my head I cried "how could they think I would harm my baby". Twenty-four years later and recounting that entire situation brings back that physical pain, the intensity lesser because, well - time, but it hurts two-fold. The memory of the suffering and also the ache to go back and hold broken 16 year old me is ever prevalent. I wish we knew then I was Autistic, so much I wish it, because as I sit here and write this, my inner child is on her knees sobbing and actual tears stream down my face once more.

And breathe.

RSD isn't always this dramatic but it is always pretty intense. As a meticulous worker with attention to detail, if a colleague or manager criticised my work then it's pretty much guaranteed I will cry. I'm not trying to manipulate the situation with "crocodile tears", I'm simply wounded, hate confrontation and feel like a fool. I cry a lot. I don't know if it's all RSD based but I can't bloody help it. I even cry when I'm angry, not just every day pissed off kind of angry but outright furious anger results in tears and I cannot stop them with all the will in the world. I cry when I'm happy, I cry when I'm proud. If you cry, I cry. Basically, I'm just a blubbering mess.

Even now as I close this chapter, I'm thinking, oh god, no-one is going to read this book and if they do they're going to realise what an absolute freak I really am. I must be coming across like such a twat. Pipe down brain.

It's ok to fucking age

Why have we been told ageing is bad?
who's idea was this farce?
memories from years gone past
and for some reason we are shocked
that we look so young then
and so old now.
well yes a decade is ten solid years.
I would not wish to be back there,
for all the money in the world.

Because ageing is growing
and understanding
and best of all,
taking less shit off other people.
having your wits about you
to finally set boundaries
and to give so many less fucks.

So cheers to ageing
the grey hairs, the years.
for they bring so much more
wealth per annum, than
any pert boob can.

Communication deficit

The irony is not lost
that in reaching out
about my inability
to communicate deeply,
for help from my therapist,
to overcome this vulnerability.

And a small stepping stone
of a solution is provided.
In theory, yes,
this sounds great
so I buy the cards
a game for ice breaker
meaningful conversations.

And they are
sat in my bag hidden.
like a figurative interpretation
of me and my mind
hidden, internalised,
safe though.

Whilst my actual mind
runs through conversations
of how I suggest we play this game
I even got as close tonight
as actually turning off the TV.

But alas the words failed me
and the cards remain hidden
their existence unknown.

Breaking the cycle

When I was 12 maybe 13
my mum put on a video
called the silent scream
a fuzzy black and white screen
of a baby in utero
as utensils entered stage left
you could see the baby retreating
mouth wide, nowhere to go.

When you were 13
I told you about the video
that scarred me for years
I told you that if you
were ever in that position
I would want to know
so that I could take you to a clinic
and hold your hand
you never have to be alone
no judgement.

I learnt about periods at school
from friends and my sisters
I was one of the last to start at school too
I remember telling my sister
when mine began
and nothing much else
was ever discussed with my mum
I remember that time
I'd already levelled up to tampons
and my sister was still scared
so I gave her a demo, using my hands
my dad used to exit the room
if my sisters and I talked about

anything period related.

When you started yours
we'd already told you all you know
I felt sad for you
"sorry poppet, that's what you'll have
every month until your 40s or 50s"
I gave you hot water bottles,
chocolate, painkillers and cuddles
because periods do hurt
and at 40 I'm still not over
having them all the bloody time
you don't have to just
put up and shut up
because they suck
and I understand
I recreate the tampon demo
with my hand
your dad will buy us tampons
and comfort food when
we have our periods.

When I was a teenager
I wasn't allowed boys in my room.
I wasn't taught about why
or consent or what things
the boys would try,
girls were allowed
with no supervision
we weren't allowed to watch
anything with gays on the television
or even a bit of romance
turn it over

When you were ten

we watched Imitation Game
you couldn't believe
it was illegal to love
who you wanted to
if their gender was the same
when you were thirteen
we watched Grey's Anatomy
and you learnt that
loving who you wanted
was normal no matter
if you were L, G, B or T.

When I was fifteen,
I went on the pill
I hid the tablets in my video player
My mum found them
and hit the roof
despite being responsible and cautious
with my boyfriend and contraception,
I was a sullied slut
and these pills were the proof.

When you were fifteen
we talked about sex
about trust and relationships
we watched Sex Education
and kept conversations open
I said when you felt it was time
I would book an appointment
and get you on something
so that you ultimately
didn't have to become a parent
before you were ready.

When I was fifteen

I liked a boy and sometimes a girl
for me I didn't see a difference,
all I knew is that I had to hide
the same sex stuff
because that was bad
and would send me to hell
I had relationships in secret
because I was taught that
they were sinful and shameful
I had to hide who I really was.

When you were thirteen
I remember you telling me
a girl at school liked you
and you didn't really like her back
not because she was a girl,
she was just a bit annoying
when you were 15 you
embraced your queer identity
and at 16 we took you to pride
and celebrated there with you.

All my life I was taught
that marriage was the aim,
that although you can't trust
boys in your bedroom,
finding one to settle down
with is the game
and you are his
and you serve him
and you must save yourself
for marriage.

We have taught you
that there are some

bad apples out there
to be wise and understand
your own vulnerability
that sex is something
to be enjoyed between
consenting people
that trust is important,
and relationship equality
emotional connection
and happiness.

You don't have to be
anyone else but you
you are incredible
just how you are
we support you
and love you
and you deserve
all the happiness
and we will always
be here to listen.

A brave day

I was brave today
and vulnerable
I spoke about things
I usually keep inside
and it was hard
but it wasn't so bad
and I will try again
someday soon,
hopefully

Go me!

What would you say?

What would you say if I told you?
if I finally plucked up the courage
to let you in on a secret neither
of us for forty years even knew?

I'm Autistic, do you know what that means?
would you care enough to find out?
not only that but I'm 90% sure
I also have ADHD.

Would you brush it off or
would you want to know more
about my new found identity?

Would it shock you to know that
all the troubles I had growing up
were not because I was a difficult child
but because of my Neurodiversity?

Because I still haven't told you
about this crucial part of me
because I'm protecting myself
from the disappointment of you
not being able to properly see.

Showering

I need a shower
my hair isn't so bad
but it doesn't feel clean enough
to fiddle with
and I hate having it tied up
but getting in the shower
means the following tasks

Getting out of my pyjamas
but it's chilly
bare feet on the cold tiles
waiting for the shower water
to be warm enough before
it can assault my skin
getting cold whilst waiting for it
icy spray catching my legs
until it's ready
stepping into the water
the good bit!
the warmth raining down on me
the steam enveloping the room
is a misty bliss

Now I don't want to do the chore
of actually washing
I don't like when shampoo bubbles
get in my ears
and the sooner I start the ritual
the sooner I have to get out
and I'm already thinking about
the cold damp air on my skin
prickling at my body hair
the laborious task of towelling dry

and still seemingly being
clammy to touch
the water in my ears when I'm
no longer in the water

Choosing what to wear for the day
whether I can moisturise
because if I don't have time for
it to fully sink in then it's a nope
because the feeling of my
sticky body in clothes is too much
do I have the energy to blow-dry
my hair, will it make me too hot

Now I don't want the clothes
I chose because I'm overheating
despite spending twenty minutes
scrolling my phone in a towel
because I picked it up to get
a look at the weather to make
and outfit decision but
forgot what I was doing

Monday Existential Crisis Day

Monday morning
existential crisis day
what do I want from my life
I just don't know anymore
unmasking layer by layer
is a confusing process
a healing process too
but who is this woman
and what the bloody hell
is she supposed to do?

Capacity Tuesday

Capacity Tuesday
today I had some extra
just a touch more
capacity to function

I got out of bed
and head to the shower
before anything could
interrupt my determination

I walked the smallest
to school, we even took her bike
I mentally noted just
two tasks for this day with
some unexpected motivation

I went straight
to my office to
tick off that first one
much to my surprise
only took an hour or so
until completion

Then I carefully
removed every cobweb
skeleton and bat
each and every single
Halloween decoration

I sifted through the fridge
gathering bits of veg
chopping up and simmering
for a soupy concoction

I have a confession
this day of dedication
from my brain is
and unexpected day of action
and possibly a one-off exception

Let down meltdown

Today was tough
being Autistic
and advocating
for yourself
is hard enough
then I find out
the four months
and two chase ups
I've done with the GP
has still ended
in my ADHD referral
being lost in the ether
why me?

Back to square one
well, it's pretty rough
I cried and sobbed
as I couldn't hold it in
why does it have
to be this way
to fight and struggle
and be let down
by the system to
get the help I
so very much need
at best is inaccessible
for those actually with ADHD
and at worst outright
triggering, traumatic
and demoralising

So we start again
back to the beginning

but she was trying her best
to support me better
I got off the phone
and cried some more
took myself to bed
put on my comfort show
whilst using a fidget toy
wow these actually work
who would have thought it
I managed to calm myself
despite it all being
a bit shit.

Inaccessibility rant

If like me you've been through the challenges of going down the NHS route for an ADHD assessment, you'll understand how monumentally frustrating it is. Wait time aside, the system is deliberately set up to deter people from attempting to get assessed. The medical secretary I spoke to (and proceeded to have a full blown meltdown to) openly admitted that it's not made easy in the hope that it sorts out the time wasters. Which of course set me right off. The irony of this approach is it's preventing the actually vulnerable ADHDers from getting the help they need. The very make up of having an ADHD brain is what prevents me from being organised enough to call them in the first place. It's what makes form filling one of my major nemesis activities. Furthermore, I had actually beyond all belief filled out their forms, emailed them and chased them a couple of times despite it being a huge and major struggle for me and still it wasn't enough. I told her so, through my sniffling, stuttering inhales and sobs.

She became a lot more helpful after this fact, which was very sweet and offered to even have me go in and she could go through the forms with me. Thanks but no thank you very much, as a self confessed hold-it-all-inner, I wasn't about to sit with a stranger and go through all my deficits (again!).

What struck me as both odd and frustrating was her insinuation that maybe I should see the GP for some "help" in the meantime. By help, I'm pretty sure (and this is an assumption) she wanted to get the crying crazy lady some medication to numb the insanity. That is not what I needed, and still do not. What I need is a relevant diagnosis and treatment for the underlying issue not for the meltdown their incompetence has caused me to have, because they "lost" my referral for four months.

Problem to be fixed

No I don't want to be fixed
I need your empathy
not your solutions

No I don't want to be fixed
I'm Autistic
I'm not sick

No I don't want to be fixed
I want a society
that is more understanding
a world that is accommodating

No I don't want to be fixed
I want to feel my emotions
no matter how big
not hide them from you
so that you aren't uncomfortable

No I don't want to be fixed

I am not broken

Society is the broken one

Fix that

Fireworks

Remember remember
the 5th of November
Also remember your
love hate relationship
with firework displays
the many you've missed
without really knowing why

The Autistic realisation
there's too many people
you never have the right
outfit or coat for the
weather and temperature
regulation situation
the queues
queues to park
queues for food and drink

Ugh the people, so many
it's cold and it's dark
probably raining too
they advertise the time
that the fireworks start
but we all know
they never do
always a delay
in the dark and the cold
surrounded by people

But when they finally begin
the lights are so pretty
and a big sensory stim
from the colours

to the crackles
and the booms that
rattle gloriously
from your head
to your bones within

A Neurodivergent family

Filling forms sucks
my attention span is waning
the focus is dissipating
so many questions
some seem the same
but worded slightly different
and of course I cannot
give brief and concise
answers to the interrogation
for fear of forgetting something
and causing a misrepresentation
of what life is like for me
an Autistic with suspected ADHD

On top of this I also need
to complete a form
for my youngest child
who masks at school
and is anxiety ridden
don't miss anything out
because at school
she keeps it all hidden

An exhausting day
of compiling our deficits
rounded off by my phone ringing
to discuss my other daughter
and the classes she's been skipping
she's gone nonverbal now
so we chat through the
notes app on my phone
I then have to compile an
email to discuss her needs

As I climb into bed
I reflect that being Autistic
with Neurodivergent kids
is equal parts wonderful
and feeling misunderstood
and alone

Never quite good enough

Never quite understood friendships
as young as four or five

Never quite focussed enough
to learn in school and thrive

Never quite patient enough
for the long winded activity

Never quite clued up enough
to understand your hostility

Never quite attentive enough
to work out your intention

Never quite disabled enough
to trigger an intervention

Never quite well behaved enough
to make you proud

Never quite brave enough
to speak my feelings aloud

Never quite good enough
to achieve what others find easy

Never quite confident enough
to simply just be me

Let me tell you something
you are enough

So change how you speak to yourself
you have learnt how to survive

You are enough
your patience has got you this far
your creativity has lead you here

You are enough
your compassion has gifted you knowledge
your growth has taught you boundaries

You are enough
so take pride in who you are
because darling you're incredible

You are enough
the world needs more people like you
so let your weird shine bright

You are enough
you've found your wonderful people
but above all you've found you
and you are the star

Befuddled Brain

My self worth is wrapped up
in my work, yet my
greatest achievements are
my beautifully kind children

My children need me
not just for the logistical and practical
side of things with the forms and pick ups
but the additional needs, the therapy
and the emotional energy

I'm focussing so much on them and
what they need, they need me
I need to be their cheerleader
and their advocate

This leaves me with not much left
because I am also dealing with
my own post diagnosis healing
so my capacity is done

Nothing left for work
which leaves me in limbo
confused about the what now
I am so proud of my business
but right now I have no capacity
to push through with it

I am so mentally and physically spent
with the phone calls
the zoom meetings, the assessments
the fighting for understanding
the hugs, the patience

the emotional support,
that there is nothing left

So when the guilt rears
it's ugly head and
takes what remaining shred is left
and I'm in the minus
my brain befuddled with
the mixed messages
and the empty battery

I love my job and my business
but I love my children more
and I need some time to learn to love me

The brain switch on

My brain just switches on
before I've even opened my eyes
I'm laying there in the light sleep
and **bing** guess who's up first
and you're in for a big surprise!

Remember that time you did that thing
yes 5 years ago, let's mull it over
overthink it and dissect it
ooh doesn't it make you cringe?!

Remember that song?
I'm not going to tell you the name
nope not the artist either
or where you last heard it
I'm just going to play it to you
on repeat and let you wonder
over and over what it is

Are you going to be any use today?
you should probably go to the gym
or maybe just a nice walk
get some chores done
yes I know it's 4am, you'll be tired now
we should let the day begin

It's 5am and you're still not back to sleep
I am brain and I am busy now
why don't you scroll your phone
just for a bit in the dark
oh and now bladder is awake too
best attend to her.

Then brain laughs as I stagger
to the bathroom, earplugs still in,
and attempt to stay partially asleep
back to bed and eye mask lowered
as my brain proceeds to list
the things I need to do this week

Wow it's 6am the alarm will sound soon
I hope I am not disturbing the husband
laying in bed next to me
so I give up and get up
take myself downstairs
quietly shuffling around the living room

Why can't I cry?

I have the overwhelming urge to cry today
it was there yesterday too
I can feel the pain inside my chest
a throb, a race, a flush of sadness
a need to sob until there's nothing left
but the tears do not fall
I'm sat here alone in my grief
my feelings quiet but physically bereft

That cry is concealed and silent
it's awareness felt invisibly
when I realise this internal torture
is a young girl, heavy with melancholy
this poor voiceless cry of the past
is troubled and misunderstood
that cry… she is me.

Grief is not linear

The amount of times I've experienced grief is too many for my 40 years on this planet. Most grief has been due to the loss of family or friends and it hurts. There is anger, confusion and heaps of pain. What is surprising is when it feels like it comes from nowhere, you think you've passed the point of it getting to you anymore, and then **wham**, right between the eyes.

I've used the term grief throughout this book a lot because it is the one thing that describes this process better than any other word. From trauma comes grief and I have lashings of trauma portions to add to the mix too, this is not my first rodeo. The problem with grief is it isn't linear. So one minute you can feel yourself feeling better, finally we're coming through this the other side. Then the next minute your inner child is in turmoil and you wish you could go back in time and hold yourself tight, rocking gently whilst whispering, "everything is going to be ok, you'll see".

The grief monster is more likely to appear when you are tired or as an Autistic when you are already overwhelmed, over stimulated and frankly exhausted, but it is not limited to those times and can catch you completely unawares. The beauty of writing down my thoughts and feelings is sometimes I don't even know where the sudden pain is conjuring from but as I begin to write it's like the letters on the page take over, spelling it out to me and I'm like "Oh I see! Hello grief, it's you".

What I am now learning is to lean into it, it's ok to feel these feelings, take stock, nurture yourself and let them be. As an avid bottler-upper, this is somewhat of a revelation on my part. The usual task of shoving those thoughts right back down and sticking a big old fat cork in the top so they can't escape is slowly but surely becoming obsolete. That box of trauma, if the lid is loose, set that moment free, and then there is no need to fight it so much.

A cautious burnout exit

Learning that burnout is a message
to my body and my mind
slow down, stop even
don't feel guilty following your needs
be the one to yourself that is kind

Do what you need to do
for recovery can be lengthy
it's so hard to describe
the feeling of utter burnout
but the recuperation as
I creep out and remember I am me

It's been three months this time
and I've just followed my needs
which is a revelation in itself
taking away the feeling of
"I'm mental" and just following
my own lead

The post diagnosis burnout
is a long a painful discovery
it is a necessity to take this time
learn to grow and to heal
a discovery of self and of identity

The burnout exit isn't an instant hit
it's a slow burn, a gradual crawl
one day you begin to realise that
you have a smidge more energy
there's less head banging that
metaphorical wall

Still take it slowly don't rush the process
baby steps, and each little win
you've worked hard to nurture your
entire new person with better understanding
and that's where the key lies herein

Be as kind to yourself now
as you would a dear friend
because your mind is your
spiritual garden of which you must
carefully, gently and lovingly tend

A pledge

I pledge to myself to always be true
to who I am in everything I do
to respect my whole self
set boundaries to better myself
and to protect my little family too

I pledge to younger me that I will continue
to educate my mind and others who
are open to learn about the struggles
and sacrifices that were made
to my self worth before we knew

I pledge to that child so many years ago
that despite her conflicts and confusions
she got us this far and I will endeavour
to be truly present and not let her pain
be in vain because now we shall glow

Dopamine delight

I really want a Crunchie
and now it's all I can think about

I'm going to have to put my
coat and shoes on and go out

because I really want to feel
that chocolate and crunch in my mouth.

T minus 2 day until my period is due

You are extraordinary

When I held you in my arms
I never knew that you would be
the gift that kept on giving
yes you brought us joy and happiness
and everything in between
one of the many things you gave
was a comprehension for the first time
in my life of who it is to be me

You see we loved your quirks
and kindness, your individuality
we knew you were going to be
as awesome as your brother
with your own twist of personality
we celebrated your uniqueness
your innocence and charm
you make us laugh and enrich
our lives, a cool and quiet calm

For without your radiant brilliance
I never would have known
that I am Autistic too
and now neither of us are alone
in learning all I could for you
I learnt about my brain too
I love how similar our traits are
because we can mutually empathise
I thank you for this gift of knowledge
you are extraordinary
my Neurodivergent surprise

The ghost of my Christmases past

Tis the season
of noisy family gatherings
people sitting in my chair
more children making mess
too many conversations at once
the TV is on too
and the cooker and the clinking glasses
and the sensory overwhelm
by the masses
your sense of injustice
is pushed to it's limits
as you listen to stories
that make you wince
you try all you can
to keep your mouth shut
but the heating is so high
it could boil your nan
why is it so hot in here
and I can't hear what
you're saying to me
because someone has
done a stuffing fart
and there's too many
of us squished on the sofa
it feels claustrophobic
and there's no room anywhere else
because the table's extended
and you smile through gritted teeth
as you don't want to be the
bah humbug but you can't breathe

The car-crash of change

The look back and reflect mode has initiated once more and the realisation my absolute lack of forbearance to change. I can categorically go back to some of my darkest days and ascertain that most were triggered by monumental changes.

Don't get me wrong, change can be good. However, even change that I have wanted has unexpectedly sent me reeling into the chasm of overwhelm and depths of despair I was neither anticipating nor prepared for. In 2017 we took a huge leap and moved down south. I had lived in Northamptonshire my entire life, everyone I knew was there, friends and family. I could probably drive the a45 and a14 with my eyes shut - I wouldn't, that would be reckless. I was happy, my business was thriving, I adored our house and village but I just didn't want to get so old and realise I had never lived anywhere else. James put on job alerts for Dorset after many conversations and trips there. We loved the idea of being closer to the sea, at the time we were literally the furthest from it in any direction. We spent so many weekends and school holidays off in our camper van chasing the need for beaches, why not move closer? I was already shooting up and down the country for photography jobs so ultimately it was down to getting the right job for the husband. Which he did and it was all systems go.

First up we had to live with my parents for three weeks until the end of term after we sold our house. Big change. Weirdly I remember even getting annoyed with the wallpaper and picture frames in the room we were staying in. I was so unreasonably frustrated with it. When we eventually hauled everything we owned plus our three kids down to our new beautiful little cottage (with it's incredible garden), I was so excited about the new adventure. Despite the excitement and loving our new home, I was pushing past all the bad feels and ignoring them. I was three and a half hours drive away from everyone I knew but absolutely loved being so close to the beach and we fell into a routine of many many beach days. The other big change was my husband's job. He was now teaching Monday to Friday, on Saturdays and some evenings every single week. I busied myself being the supporting wife and mother whilst he settled into his new extra obligations. At the same time I was throwing myself into relocating my business, although I've always travelled far and wide for work, I really wanted to hone it in on the South West. Our youngest was now going to a childminder in the village and I was hyper focussed on a rebrand, new website and picking up as much work as I could.

The 2018 wedding season was one of my best yet but it took its toll and the cracks began to show. I was exhausted (burnout!). My mental health started to decline and I wasn't telling anyone either, just plastering on a fake smile and soldiering on whilst internalising it all. All of which contributed to my loneliness and isolation that I was already feeling. By early 2019 I found a local therapist because I couldn't stop my busy mind constantly berating myself. I could not understand why I felt this way, on the outside it looked like everything was going so well, what was wrong with me? Surely this is normal life, everyone has work and kids, husbands and houses to look after, why was I finding it all so bloody difficult?

With the move came more change than just the obvious, like what on earth do we do at Christmas now? I felt invaded with visitors and it was so confusing because I missed them but after they left, I was completely broken from the hosting, entertaining and well, just having people in my home. Living far away meant that there was no easy way to do it without either; being away from the safety of my own home or having them in it for multiple days because no-one wants to do a 7 hr round trip in a day. Christmas Day 2019 I will never forget bawling silently in the bath with everyone downstairs and intrusive thoughts of what if I just plunged myself underwater and drowned to stop it all. Of course I could never act on it, imagine having the ruining of Christmas forever as my parting gift to my loved ones. Why is everything so hard for me, I just couldn't fathom any other reason than I must be useless, broken and it was my fault.

When the world stopped in March 2020 something switched inside me. Yes I was still dealing with the trauma of it all, especially my business which is wrapped up in my self worth. But the actual slowing down was like a breath of fresh air, I could breathe again. Probably not the best analogy given the very make up of the pandemic but I was gifted time and I felt a sense of relief. I couldn't work, I couldn't have people come and stay. I had our son Jake and his girlfriend live with us for three months during the first lockdown as literally days before the shutdown of life as we knew it, I was tanking it up the m5 to collect them so they weren't stuck in University halls. Don't get me wrong, I was still manically trying to keep everyone safe and happy, coming up with wild ideas of entertainment, braving the supermarket in PPE to keep them all fed, but the time, oh the time.

The pottering in the garden, the silly games, we even did a vow renewal in the garden for our wedding anniversary on 26th April 2020, so wholesome. We had time to workout, run, walk, read. The community camaraderie in the village was exceptional too. With further regulations and more lockdowns it was apparent I was going to have to suck it up and get a key worker job, because not only that, due to being a LTD company, I had exactly zero financial support from the Government. I ended up working at a school during lockdown 2 or was it 3, I can't keep up. My colleagues were amazing but the circumstances were weird and my whole life felt confusing as fuck. It wasn't long before I was in burnout again. Sometimes the burnout was mentally obvious, and others even my body broke down for the ride. I still didn't know I was Autistic and I was still forcing myself to get up and carry on.

I would like to add a disclaimer here, about the seriousness of the global pandemic and how it has affected everyone. I know I was happy with the gift of time in the early days but I am also wholly aware of all the people that died and the lives that were and still are being ruined. We lost my Mother-in-law in November 2021 and my husband couldn't even enter the hospital until the worst was feared and imminent. His last conversations with his mum were over the phone and covid kept him from her.

It takes me and my brain an excruciatingly long time to process change and trauma, and as I sit here typing, I'm still not "over" the pandemic.

Trust my boundaries

Trust that my boundaries
are there to serve me
not to inconvenience you

Trust that they have
been put in to place
after decades of having none

A boundary is an example
of my growth
after years of believing
the problem is me

Don't push my boundary
for once it is broken
so too will the trust be
between you and I

Trust my boundaries
for they protect my wounds,
my soul, my present and my future

My boundaries are indispensable
sometimes temporary
and others are forever

Trust my boundaries
and I will reciprocate
with trust in you

Toxic validation seeker

I hope that you read that title as it came out of my brain onto this page and if you are of a certain age you will understand "Secret Lemonade Drinker"

Growing up, I never belonged
I felt unwanted and shunned,
by my peers, my teachers, my family
it was apparent I never could
get anything quite right

I had friends but always felt
low on the friendship hierarchy
outside looking in at the
best friends that I would
never be able to attain

So I sought validation
wherever I could find it
I moulded and bended
to fit a new narrative
lets see if this version lands

When puberty hit the
validation seeking went
dangerously into hyper drive
I medicated myself
with alcohol and drugs
a wonder I managed to survive

I discovered as my body
grew and developed
I actually did have something
that some people wanted

and I used it for that forever
wanted validation high

I've lost count of the
perilous situations
my toxic validation seeking
has lead me to be in
the risks, jeopardy and instability

It was no revelation that
at just 16, I fell pregnant
a curveball to my spiralling
toxic behaviour
an unplanned surprise
but a saviour no less and I'll tell you why

Becoming a mother
at just 17 years old
was a shock to my system
but a glorious dawning
began to unfold

For this baby boy
taught me something
I felt I had never deserved before
taught me of unconditional love
that despite my faults I was worthy

I had a new story now
and this chapter was motherhood
and although there was still
so much to learn
it was the beginning of truth

I will be honest here now

and say I was still pretty vulnerable
a young undiagnosed single mother
easy prey for abuse

But I fought all the
labels, the teenage mum stereotype
to provide him with a good life
and in doing so eventually
I worked through my own

I often think where I might
be now if it wasn't for my son
there was still years of
validation seeking but
with a touch less risk

For I was responsible
for a whole other human now
and over the years I would
adapt, learn and grow

The validation that enriches
me these days
is seeing what an incredible
young man this baby boy
has grown up to be

For despite my sadness,
my loneliness and feeling so outcast
I created this human
I've chosen a better path
and had someone, something
to be proud of at last

Bang on brand

There is no surprise
I love and am exceptionally good
at my own marketing
I've been unknowingly,
subconsciously building my own brand
my entire life
yes this changes through the years
the jobs and relationships
the masking and mirroring

My social and professional
groups, shaping and influencing
my brand as I cultivate
the person I want the world
to know and to see
is a reflection of the person
I believe society wants me to be

Stripping back that mask
that meticulously curated brand
and working out who I really am
is daunting yet liberating
taking time to work on my
own core values in life
what is important and what is not
accepting my new unmasked self
confidently letting go of the
things and people that
no longer serve or appreciate
the truest version of me.

Where have all the safe foods gone?!

It's lunchtime again
I open the fridge
then the cupboard
and repeat
the food is all still the same
as if by some miracle
it has changed when
I reopen each door

I am bored of food
but I need to eat
I cancelled the Gousto
because well
executive function
and I couldn't bear
looking at the sad
not very fresh
ingredients any more

Rest & Remove

Rest
remove your obligations
your deadlines and invitations

Rest
remove the demands
conserve the energy life commands

Rest
remove uncomfortable clothes
listen to music and play your favourite shows

Rest
remove the guilt and shame
charge your power to reclaim

The pieces of me

Am I hypochondriac
or do I just feel too much
not just the emotions
but the pieces of me too

I can feel when the smallest
of hairs on my arm moves
it's like tiny creatures
inching across my skin

The washing machine belly
I so lovingly named
for that fast spin can often
wake me in the middle of the night

My ovary is aching,
I know when it expels
another potential for procreation
a waste of time dear ovary
don't even get me started on menstruation

I twist and turn my ankles
to stretch them out
after a day of use
because they ache and are
as grouchy as me

The big light is way too bright
makes me feel too heady
and squinty, my poor eyes
don't like to drive at night

Is that a lump or

just normal lumpy breasts
I'll poke it for a while
until I can't think about
anything else.

My wrists hurt
and my knees
I remember my knees
misery even as a child

My heart is thumping
so loud sometimes
I can feel it beating
sometimes skipping
and worse still racing

The intense fatigue
why so tired
you've barely done a thing
but anything you
do manage is exhausting

My ears itch deep within
I can feel my eardrums
and know when they
are being stretched thin

I will confess
I am so used to every
slight, every pain
but also used to keeping
it all to myself

So late at night I
will research the possibilities

which result in thyroid,
cancer, ovarian cysts
or diabetes

Occasionally when they
have reached an absolute peak
I will book an appointment
just in case, to have my
bloods tested

All these years of extra worry
for all the pieces of me
when could it actually simply be
interoception hypersensitivity

Because I cannot concentrate
on anything else if I'm
hungry or need the bathroom
in fact it can be so stressful
if I don't meet these needs
extremely soon

The meltdowns and shut downs
that have occurred
because my body cannot
tune out of the signals
that are screaming from inside

You look nice

She compliments me on my outfit
and I graciously accept the kind words
for I was awake early hours overthinking
the perfect outfit for the social event

I did not want to wear the wrong thing
for fear of judgment and also
I still kind of wanted to look like me

I didn't want to make a wardrobe faux pas
and despite wearing my autistic friendly
ensemble for months now
I actually donned some jeans
a smart shirt, casual trainers
and some of my alternative jewellery

She complimented me on my outfit
and after a thank you I froze
as she began to chatter and smile
because am I supposed to say
something back now or will
it just be an empty courtesy

For it feels like it would be a reaction
to her endorsement of my
carefully constructed costume

In my mind she will know I didn't
come to this admiration alone
and it's forced, contrived, insincere
so I stand there like a plum
homage to her attire
I guess there will be none.

I don't think she noticed but
I have no idea what she said since

It's been several hours now
I'm tucked up in bed post social
and I lay here overthinking once more
did I miss the etiquette?!
my social ineptitude making me wince

Dutch courage, social crutch

I remember hitting my last birthday
wow the last year in my thirties
what do I want to achieve
before the big four-oh

I sat and I deliberated
what would truly bring me happiness?
unsure of where to start
I began with what does not bring me joy

Hangovers
people pleasing
social awkwardness
FOMO
dickheads

Hangovers, ok is this it?
is it time to finally say goodbye
my trusty glasses of confidence
are we really going to quit?

I went months without a drop
to see if I actually could stop
I had many a fun congregation
and trained my brain
to finally realise I didn't need
booze enabled jollification

Another year on and where are we?
well I am drinking but less binging
more of a share a bottle of wine
than lets get one each

Less need to drink just
because it's the weekend
pondering now if I can
is it possible to cut ties
with my inebriating friend

She is toxic but enticing
and even a slight lubrication
in an awkward social situation
has got to be better than when
we didn't know how to stop
once the lid had popped

I honestly wish I had the courage

The misadventure of employment

The Office Of National Statistic (ONS) reported in 2020 that a mere 22% of Autistic adults are in any kind of employment. Let's just set aside that this statistic is based on diagnosed adults which we already know there is a huge disparity especially in women and people of colour. I'm honestly not surprised because so many jobs are inaccessible or damaging to Autistic people.

My own career was propelled by my ADHD in so many ways. I literally think I am capable of most things and will give anything a bash. I had my first child when I was just 17 years old and having already grown up with many, many labels, being a scrounging teenage mum wasn't another one I wanted to add to the pile. So when my son was a year old I went to work. First was working in childcare at a nursery whilst doing an NVQ. Well did you know that apparently there's a right and wrong way to get qualifications and going down the NVQ route was seen as beneath my colleagues, who had done it the "right" way. This automatically made an unwritten hierarchy I was oblivious to. Especially considering I was actually really good at my job and some of them were not. Working with the children was really rewarding, especially helping the shy, anxious ones come out of their shell, but I couldn't stomach the toxic environment. Why do these people all moan to each other about each other all the time?! So I left.

With absolutely no idea what I wanted to do I fell into a customer service role. Responding to complaint emails seemed to be a skill I possessed and I could expertly mirror people over the phone, match their tempo, pronunciation and sometimes even their accent. All of which bode well with our customers, they seemed to like it. Around 6 months into the job I became increasingly irritated with hierarchy (again). The office manager really thought she was something special but didn't seem to work too hard to accolade herself with such privilege. I always found it weird the way people changed when she swanned into the room, talking about her "Mitsubishi Shogun" rather than just saying "car". People were constantly confusing me. Time for a change, impulsivity made me do it. I quit without another job to go to.

I was aimlessly wandering the high street, looking in shop windows at adverts, hoping for inspiration for what might be my next job. Sadly the careers advice we had at school back in the day was useless, it was a very clunky and terrible computer automated questionnaire, I think I got carpet fitter. All the girls at school either went into teaching and childcare or the lesser academically gifted went into beauty and hairdressing. So here I am, pounding the pavements questioning my life choices once again when someone hands me a leaflet for a recruitment drive for a new big IT company locally. Result!

It was an odd experience because they were recruiting for all levels of jobs. I was 20 years old, undiagnosed and a semi-expert masker by now. I remember feeling quite wanted as managers from the different departments tried to pitch jobs to me. I went with telemarketing - dishing out offers and updating the database sounded pretty simple. There was a routine to the day and I'm good at doing the phone thing, I knew that from my last role. The job was a doddle and there were ways to earn commission so that was a win for me. I learnt quite a lot on human behaviour in this role, as it was a big company with large teams in an open plan environment, plenty of opportunity for people watching. For reasons unbeknown to me, I seemed to rub some people up the wrong way. Turns out if you are young, not offensive to look at, and good at your job, some people just don't like you. I also felt like a form of prey to the older guys in the office, I can't tell you how many times I was left feeling sick and uneasy by them. I could also see them practically salivating over other young female members of staff, even the married men, drooling and being what I thought was so goddamn obvious. Not obvious to everyone as it seems. Studying human interactions has made me cautious but also a pretty accurate judge of character. It got tiresome and the 6 month ants-in-my-pants began. Technology had become interesting to me though, it just made sense, so I looked for another IT company maybe a little closer to home. Oh and there was the fact that I was scared I was about to lose my driving license as I got caught with no insurance. Hear me out! ADHD tax; I simply forgot to do my renewal, actually no that's not quite true, I called to renew and they didn't take my bank card (hands up if you remember the Natwest Solo debit cards, useless things) and I forgot to call them back. A new job that I could walk to would be good, just in case.

Somehow I had upgraded to a full sales role at a different IT company. The training was my favourite bit; I got to spend hours in the service department with the geeks learning about the components that made a computer work. My brain was like a sponge absorbing it all. All I had to do now was build up my own customer base and sell the components to them. A challenge I could rise to with my conversation scripting skills. I'd gone from one extreme to the next.

Huge open plan, noisy, busy, wall-to-wall windows to a dreary and windowless office in a warehouse. Not a fan, but it was a means to an end. The masking and mirroring again came in very handy when building a rapport with clients. I could be whoever they wanted me to be and from previous human studying I learnt that "knowledgeable with an edge of flirty" with IT managers was the route to my commission. Evidently I could only keep this shit up for 6 month stints until I needed to shake it up and leave. One day I took a message for a colleague from one of their customers and boredom had me idly looking up the company online. I thought it looked pretty cool for a place of work. Another IT company but less selling IT parts and more selling entire products and solutions. Their offices looked like a decent middle ground to the job I was in and my previous job. So I just waltzed right in there one day in my lunch break and asked to speak to the Manager, told him I wanted a job there and got myself an interview.

This place would be where I met my now husband but it wasn't all sweetness and roses. I'm still undiagnosed at this point and there are many, many things causing me grief that I don't understand. Although my comprehension of hierarchy is much improved I still don't buy into it. There's one other sales woman in the office, the rest are all men so ole masky-mirror-pants over here becomes one of the lads. The company provide loads of on-going training and my Autistic brain is lapping it up like an excited puppy. The work hard, play hard theme throughout means lots of socials and my old friend alcohol brings out party Hannah that everyone seems to like. I'm sure the Directors would have called it like a "family" but it was not far off cult like in those early days. As long as you were putting in your hours (and not first to leave) and spending all your hard earned money down the pub with them then you were "in". I actually felt like I belonged somewhere for the first time in a long time but it was not to last. More on that in a bit.

The company grew a lot in the time I was there, new things happened like new seating arrangements (shudders from school days) and I did not like change much, especially if it meant that someone who chewed their pen constantly (Misophonia), inhaled packets of salt and vinegar crisps and hated women sat next to me. I was burning out and didn't know it. By 3pm most days I was struggling to work through sheer exhaustion, maybe it was the partying, or maybe the antihistamine (except it wasn't happening in winter too). I couldn't regulate my body temperature and it was a running joke how many times I would take my jacket on and off through the course of the day. I had headaches (fluorescent lights) I would list my symptoms to colleagues and they would suggest I get my bloods done for Diabetes or Thyroid and I agreed, well there are Thyroid issues in the family. I can't tell you how many times I've had my bloods tested over the years wondering what is wrong. Newsflash - I was over stimulated, over whelmed and burning out.

After having Erin (and being treated awfully as the first sales woman to have a baby I might add), we stopped going out with work like we used to, which I presumed was a normal thing when you become parents. The social etiquette of office politics and playtime was evident. We no longer belonged and were dropped from the inner circles of the cult, I mean office. We still went out occasionally but there was a marked difference in how people behaved with me. I never forget being told I was intimidating by one of the managers which blew my mind as I'd spent years, working very hard on being a friendly person.

The biggest red flag to my autism in the workplace was exactly when I knew I needed to get out (but still didn't know about my Neurodivergence). The London riots were happening, I'd spent all night watching the news absolutely bereft and worried sick about our friends in the area and well, society in general. As I got into work that morning one manager was hell bent on bullying the interns about it. He went on and on, somehow blaming them for the London riots just because they were young. Yep you guessed it, social injustice warrior woman reared her head (that's me) and I slammed him down (with words, I am small and weak!). I could see the whole office too scared to stick up for the young men whilst simultaneously shocked by the manager's behaviour, why was no-one backing me on this. Then he started this annoying high-pitched ranting and general noise making. To me it felt like several sharp, pokey things stabbing me in the brain and ears, I actually physically felt it and he just wasn't stopping. I shouted, "Can you stop? it's making me feel stabby". Which of course went exceptionally well - no it did not. I can't remember exactly what happened next but I walked out. Put in an official complaint to HR about it and refused to come back until it was dealt with.

The more senior manager asked to meet with me outside of work so I dutifully went. What I wasn't expecting, was to be told the bully manager had put in a counter complaint to HR, saying that I threatened to stab him. It was a mess, I felt awful that someone could lie like that to try and save themselves. In what felt like a matter of weeks, he was promoted to the senior team and well I jumped ship completely. Fuck that.

During this time I had been throwing myself into the hobby/hyper-focus of photography and was actually studying it at night college so this seemed like the right time to just go for it and that's exactly what I did. I set up my own business, worked from home by myself with full control over my environment and what people I let into my sphere. It was flipping amazing. Like anything, there are still challenges, however, I could meet my needs myself and turns out I'm pretty bloody good at this photography lark. The longest I've stuck at anything, 11 years and counting.

Empathy Curse

I am told I am blunt
intimidating even
I don't mince my words
she says it exactly how it is

I cannot hide if your
new haircut looks shit
or the idea you had
was weak I'll admit

But if I see your sadness
I will completely crumble
I will take on that pain
the torment is humble

Physically and emotionally
I feel it all under my skin
the destruction and injustice
my heartache begins

I cry at the hopelessness
the state of our earth
each infringement, transgression
becomes even worse

The news is switched off
because I can't bear all the fight
as I lie trapped in my mind
the grief stealing my night

The pain of my loved ones
even strangers too
can be so deep and intense

oh the empathy, if only you knew

Yes I'm Autistic
and my perceptions diverse
but trust me they penetrate
with this empathy curse

Evangelical bralette pusher

It's funny when you look back
maybe not even that far
and realise your autistic need
for a revolution of the trusty bra

I remember around 2017
the Saviour of my big breasts
at last someone has thought of us
my rib cage can finally rest

When I discovered the bralette
I couldn't keep it to myself
I don't know how I've worn these
wired bras my whole boobed life

So I told all my friends thinking
every tittied person should know
they tried mine on as we laughed
at the ridiculous bra show

But look these are comfy
I have bought them all
I know I'm evangelical but
your boobs can be comfy
even if they're not small

The slug and pillow

In the past my family believed
I was a little bit hard of hearing
but it turns out I just can't
concentrate on processing
audio with all the other
sounds interfering

If the TV is on and the radio
in the other room too
I cannot understand
the words coming from you
If I'm writing an email
or reading some text
I cannot hear your words
or your simple request

But remember that time
I said the pillow was loud
you looked at me weird
and said it makes no sound
I'll never forget that night
I was trying to sleep on the sofa
there was a slug on the floor
and I could hear the damn thing
each time it inched closer

If like me you see pub signs, band names and t-shirt slogans all the time... this poem title is one of those times, you're welcome.

Unmasking acceptance

Thank you my friends for
being the awesome humans you are
for accepting my diagnosis
for understanding
for empathising
for wanting to know more
I love you dearly
I will forget to text you back
or forget what day it is
and subsequently your birthday
but I will be there for you
as you are for me
and I'm pretty damn good
in a crisis emergency

Fight, flight and freeze

Forty years of survival mode
fight, flight and freeze
fuck

So flighty

As a child I ran away
I never got very far
I ran away because
of my executive dysfunction
and really physically couldn't
tidy my room
I ran away because
of my rejection sensitivity
not handling your criticism
I ran away because
I felt like I simply
didn't belong
I ran away because
I felt like no-one
understood me
I ran away from school
because my needs
weren't being met
I ran away in my mind
pondering if you would
care if I didn't exist

Well shit, I'm disabled

I am disabled
this is a an actual fact
though hard it seems
to actually get my
head around

Autism isn't an excuse
for all my battles
it is a reason
a reason as to why
those challenges
have been a never ending
up hill struggle
often ending in failure

Even in my successes
the trials and tribulations
to actually achieve
were monumental
and in turn my successes
are greater than
I originally imagined

Acknowledging my disability
does not come easy
but it certainly makes it
all make sense.

A need to know basis

When I ask you the plans
it's not because I don't like them
or because I want to take control
it's a process of understanding
so that I can prepare myself
to prepare for timings
to avoid the time meltdown
to pre-empt the situation
or subsequent over stimulation
to plan for sensory issues that may arise
so there isn't unexpected overwhelm
from a last minute surprise.

Finding her Autistic voice

Is she acting more Autistic
now that she has a diagnosis
or has she simply
found her Autistic voice
for she can tell you now
what she needs

100% Autistic

Who me? Yes.

Unmasking is not to be taken lightly. The imposter syndrome is so strong some days it's hard to ignore. Am I acting more Autistic since my diagnosis and unmasking journey? 100% I am. Folding back the tired old mask(s) means not holding back and hiding who I am anymore. There's been so many times since July that I've just been like "who even am I?" But slowly, softly, like David Attenborough describing a rare bird in the rainforest, whilst also trying not to alert said bird and scare it off, I'm discovering who was locked up inside for so long.

I'm not quite there yet with showing the entire world - yes I've written a book, but as I currently type, this book is just here and not yet **there**, *motions to big wide world with an outstretched arm.* I'm more unmasked at home than anywhere else. I am more "me" around my close friends (weirdo magnet) and my sister because they get it. I am at my most Autistic when I'm alone, (this might sound obvious) but I have had to also unmask to myself. Flapping and clapping my hands with joy is a regular occurrence now whilst the house is empty. Talking to myself, dancing, swaying, stimming, repeating words aloud that I like, the cat thinks I am positively bonkers (spoiler; I am!). Previously I was writing to do lists and mostly getting so frustrated with myself about why I could never achieve things in a day like a "normal" person. Constantly berating myself for being useless. Now I'm embracing the low energy days of rest as much as the high-energy days of productivity, they are both valid.

The noise cancelling headphones that James bought me have got to be the most wonderful aid to my autism ever. Asking him for them took a lot of courage and I had to fight my own internalised ableism. It felt too cliché to have them as an Autistic person but once I wrestled that nagging bear to the ground and got what I needed, just wow. I was already wearing earplugs to bed every night and have some day time ones to lower decibels in busy places like shopping, restaurants or *shudders* kids parties. The noise cancelling headphone-cans are just another level. I can listen to music, podcasts or brown noise whilst doing anything from housework, to computer work. I use them to block out Mila's cartoons, she needs them to decompress after school and I need to not hear them after a long day, except now we can exist in the same room together with both our needs being met. I even had them on with some music whilst reading the other night because James was fidgeting with something whilst he was reading and who am I to over-rule a need to move/stim. The gym, the supermarket, the school run, the uses are endless and liberating as fuck.

It's not all revelations and rainbows. Presenting more Autistic also makes me realise just how much of a people-pleasing zombie I was before. I rarely voiced my needs until it was too late and I was having a meltdown that I could no longer avoid. This means that now I'm unmasking, I feel like I am being more demanding (shush Hannah, it's called setting boundaries). The post diagnosis burnout is so long, just when I think - this is it, I realise it is not. Honestly I'm not sure if I'll ever feel like I did before. This listening to my body and mind lark has made me realise just how debilitating being Autistic can be, how on earth did I make it this far in life without having a breakdown? Oh yeah, that's right, I didn't. Breakdowns I might add, that I kept to myself, I waded through that pain alone because I was too scared that my loved ones would run for the hills if they really knew what went on inside my head.

The beauty of being more authentic to myself and others is the worst of my brain struggles can actually be nipped in the bud before it escalates. Sure sometimes I still need to shutdown and not speak when I'm overwhelmed but that's ok.

Hugh Jackman shimmies across the stage and belts out "This is Me" à la the Greatest Showman

Burden

Am I a burden?
or is my internal monologue
an ableist little shit?

Local derby

There is a local derby
inside my head
it's a match between
my autism and my ADHD

Although yes there
are many similar things
with both teams
they compete against
each other too

Autism: let's plan
and structure everything
ADHD: let's do
something spontaneous
Autism: I'm happy at home
ADHD: let's go socialise
Autism: I need clarity
and organisation
ADHD: I'm going to
wing it, it will be messy

In wades the task paralysis
and the executive dysfunction
with it's size 12 boots
wiping out the pitch
and now no-one can play

The witches and the weirdos

I can't help but feel
that those burned at the stake
tried as witches
thrown in asylums
were our Neurodivergent sisters
mistaken, not conforming
the disobedient, fidgety girls
unable to be married off
hidden away
to circumvent family shame
the spinsters and
the cat ladies
the alternative thinkers
the "hysterical" women
the creative tinkers
I often think about you all

Do not disturb

Burnout hot tip
for you my friend
I left my phone on DND
for 3 days solid
5/5 would recommend

Although I did miss the text about gammon from the husband until he phoned me from Morrisons (he is on the privileged list for calls to come through).

Bumps

As I buffed and polished
my nails today
she asked what does it do
so I showed her my hand
that has been done and
the hand that had not
she rubbed her tiny finger
across the opposing nails
the before and the after
the faulty and fixed
see this one is smooth
and this one is bumpy
do mine she asks
I begin to work the surface
of her flawless, dainty thumb nail

Finished… feel it? can you see?
Oh she says
I wanted the bumps

We can learn a lot from a 6 year old

The mind of a 6 year old is such a wonderful place to be. Imagine not being swayed by society and the media about what is wrong and what is right. Finding the beauty in imperfections.

I watch Mila and I'm like wow kid you are so flipping incredible. You take her to the beach and she will find beauty in a rock, it's just a rock, but look Mum it has this cool spot on it, or this hole or this rough bit. She will bounce up and down on a yoga ball solidly for an entire movie, no shits given about what she looks like, she is just loving the movement. Talks to any stranger, especially if they've got a nice hat "I like your hat".

The Saturday morning, self-chosen outfit combos are my favourite. She's not interested in anything scratchy but that little human dopamine-dresses like a champ. Some days it's tutus and a tail, the next could be declared a PJ or onesie day (citing the "my body, my choice" I taught her when she was 3). Alternatively it's a pants-on-her-head day (well why not).

In the summer she raised her own caterpillars to butterflies, honestly I did not know how it would go when we got to the setting them free part. But as she carefully coaxed each one from the enclosure, the delight on her face as she spoke softly to them, encouraging them to fly - *heart melt*. She turned to me and said it made her happy to see them take off in the sunshine.

At a firework display, I looked on in total awe and respect as among hundreds of people, Mila started to dance in a small clearing on her own. Her body was popping and jumping along to the music and the bangs of the fireworks. She was the only one and she was exhilarated in her own world just feeling the moment and letting her body do as it pleased.

The wonder of the mind of a 6 year old is out and out glorious and I implore you all to seize the day like a child, find your joy and heal your inner child in the process. I've just treated myself to a new pair of roller skates, I never stopped skating as a child. As an adult I've done it on and off over the years and after a hiatus I always think, why haven't I done this in so long. It is utter joy. I even braved a skate park recently, during the school day so it was empty – I'm not completely mad. Swishing around that park was so freeing and hit all the right sensory seeking and dopamine high spots. Up with this sort of thing.

More goddamn forms

How do I do even more
the questions the same
but more in-depth
specific examples
of my ADHD traits in childhood
but I don't remember much
no I don't still have
my school reports of
yesteryear
I'm 40 for fuck sake
yes I am up in the middle
of the night
frantically typing notes
into my phone
because I can't sleep
and I'm going through
the filing system
of my brain
like someone looking for
clues to a mystery
in the office of a suspect
it's dark outside
there is a torch surreptitiously
dangling between my teeth
as I scan each folder
for the facts and evidence

Failure

Sometimes I just wake up
feeling like a failure

12 hours

It took me a solid
12 hrs to get
into a bath today
and 2hrs to get
back out again
straight back
into pyjamas
hair still wet
because there
is nothing left
for the palaver
of drying it
I am clean and
I've got a baileys though
the little wins
Christmas Eve tomorrow!

Hair bobble

I tried to go an extra stretch
another day without a hair wash
because my day was focused,
focused on food timings
and not forgetting any of the menu
with a household of complex palettes
and different food needs
(dinner was banging by the way)
the day was chill with
no unwanted surprises
I even had time out to read
with my headphones on

Then out of nowhere
came an un-ignorable ick
with my goddamn hair
my go-to style is down
as I can't bear the tightness
of it up and restricted
but all of sudden the stress
that this hair ick did
was all I could think of
as I searched high and low
for a very specific scrunchie
it's velvet and not so tight
I could not find it
not even a decent replacement
in any flipping sight

I settled on a random
scrunchie with a stupid bow
thankfully the sensory ick was over
and although I was expressing

my distress I didn't enter
a full blown meltdown
later that evening Erin
came to me with two
little hair bobbles
for next time and
a nod of understanding

The closing of a year

An unease deep within me
as we near the closing
of the year once more

It's almost impossible
not to reflect on what the
last 365 days has been

I know it's human to think
of all the things that
have brought pain

As the first few thoughts
slow dance to the
forefront of my brain

Delicate but deliberate
as they oscillate
teasing my emotions

Because I know once
I succumb to this
memory invitation

The steps will be
reflexive as they
tentatively spiral

Pull me down to
a sad place where
I will dance alone

So this time as we

near the closing
of another year

I will stand up
up the tempo
ignore the sorrowful proposal

With a change in direction
and new choreography
I will let my limbs shake wild

Wild with joy
because look at us now
look what we have

An awakening of self
as I leap into the
wonder of my brain

Close my eyes and feel
the rhythm of the good
vibrating into my soul

Dancing to the beat
of my own happiness

Shedding the weight

This January I'm shedding the weight
the weight of other people's expectations
for they are not worthy of my worry

I see your diet ads and your exercise fads
and I raise you, self belief
and the weightlessness of not being
controlled by a number on the label
of my clothes (of which I've cut out, itchy things)
or the scales on which
I'm probably not going to stand on

The heaviest thing I have carried
for the longest of time is the narrative
that I am worthless unless I fit into the
MO of self-deprecation, of "naughty" foods
and the constant (very boring) chat
of "being good" this year

I am good, I am kind, and I am working
on my true authentic self
none of which is dictated by what
I put on my back or nourish my body with

Not my first rodeo

Not my first rodeo and other
sayings that enter my repertoire
each building on my scripted
conversations for social situations
the times in primary school
when I enjoyed new words
teased for my use of humid (a lot)
turns out is a product of
an autistic trait called echolalia

Sometimes it's an instant repetition
most times it's one for the word bank
as I repeat it over and over in my mind
thinking about how I like it
I loved a thesaurus to discover new words
having felt different, stupid even
I used them to try and be better
to be accepted as more intelligent

I am fierce

When I was little I was not fierce
I had my quirks and my innocence
I was a bit of a joker and I loved to play
I had my own little worlds of joy
growing up I realised I didn't fit in anymore
this was still my personality
as others got older I was misunderstood
left out and bullied constantly

I masked that girl
stripped that innocence away
now she was tough, small but mighty
she would challenge anyone who
attempted to do her a disservice
she got loud and vocal about each slight
she changed schools to flex her
new main character

Though on the outside she was fierce
inside she got even lonelier
so unbelievably vulnerable
she found herself in many a scary
situation with zero protection
given up on by teachers and parents
no genuine friends to come to her aid
nothing left but to work out herself
how to break free from the mess
of a bed that she had in fact made

The can do and the cannots

I can turn my hand to most things
I will try and build, make, craft
write, create, make a business from scratch

I cannot organise my home, tidy consistently,
meal plan, remember important things
find my keys, sort out my clothes,
know where my phone is, when it's in
my actual hand

I can fight injustice, raise an army to join me,
talk at length and passionately
about the things I am interested in
I cannot do the small talk

I can hand stencil my bathroom floor
over 2 days for a combined total
of 14 hours non stop
but please don't make me queue
in a busy shop

Letter in my head

I woke up at 4am and began a letter in my head
of the conversations I couldn't speak to your face
but the words went unsaid

I had the chance and I had the time
I just couldn't get these words out of this
overthinking brain of mine

So as I woke in the early hours my mind began
to compose a heartfelt letter and
organising an autistic coming-out plan

Whether this actually happens I have no clue
but for now I'll start to write and maybe
just maybe I might give this letter to you

I'm sorry

I'm so sorry it may feel like
I couldn't trust you enough to talk to you

I built it up in my mind and couldn't escape
the fear and the worry of the rejection
I am so used to receiving

40 years undiagnosed, navigating the world
alone in my own head has been
detrimentally confusing

The generational gap between us
leaves a lot of room for disagreement and denial
I needed to sit on my diagnosis for a while

The letter

In for a penny in for a pound (WTF does that even mean?! It's ok, I've googled it, and it works). I figured I've bared enough of my soul by now and wouldn't it be great to include the letter I frantically typed up to my parents at the early hours. Yes, yes it would. We live 175 miles from one another, it's been nearly 6 months since my diagnosis and I've been unable to tell them. Mostly due to self-preservation and fear of rejection stopping me from doing so. Also I've been working so hard on the imposter syndrome and the validation, I was too scared to put it out there to a couple of pensioners (albeit my doting pensioner parents) who had vastly different upbringings to me, from a generation of naughty kids and discipline. I didn't want to have all my hard work being undone if they were to turn around and invalidate it all. I built it up in my head, their response and it wasn't going to be easy. However I'd also spent some time avoiding prolonged time with them because Autism is my current all consuming special interest so it would crop up if I wasn't careful, best not to see or speak to them for too long until I've worked out some shit for myself. Alas, the Christmas festivities began. Mum and Dad were coming down in the New Year and this was my time to tell them.

The husband with his ever-comedic tension slicing wit states "I'm not sure you're ready yet, and also whether we can afford the therapy afterwards" as I admitted to him on the last night of their stay what my intentions were (that I had so far failed!) of coming out as Autistic to them.

Buckle up, it's a long one

This is a huge thing for me to open up to you because it leaves me feeling extremely vulnerable and I've spent the majority of my life hiding it all, it's what I'm used to doing. I tried repeatedly to tell you this last couple of days, however the words and conversations formed in my mind and never left my mouth!

Remember when we were going through those challenges with Erin, I was talking to you on FaceTime about it and Mum you said "but you were like that".

Well when we finished the long process of Erin's autism assessment. I had connected a lot of dots for me too. I wasn't aware of how autism presented in girls but now I'm the expert on it!! A lot of what was happening with Erin just seemed "normal" to me as she is very similar to me. I didn't know it at the time but Neurodiversity is a result of genetics (or sometimes trauma at birth or an infectious disease). Therefore having an Autistic daughter there's a high chance that either James or I or both of us are also Neurodivergent.

I too have been diagnosed as Autistic back in July. I did so much research to try and support Erin I managed to unravel so much about myself I never knew. (Autism in girls & women is now one of my special interests!). The reason I have gone undiagnosed until I was 40 years old is because all autism research is done on little boys, the criteria for diagnosis is based on those studies and has thus led to a huge disparity in girls being diagnosed when young.

I am also what is known as a "high-masker" which means I internalise a lot of struggles, I masked my autism to fit in and yet never felt like I belonged anywhere…. Hence the small fortune I've paid for therapy as an adult! It is really damaging to my wellbeing to mask. I've spent the last 5 months in what is known as "Autistic Burnout" since my diagnosis because it is a snowball of processing my entire life with this new information. I've learnt that I'm not crazy which is what I've told myself many times over the years and that autistic burnout happens when I'm overwhelmed either emotionally or sensory triggered and that I am in fact not having a mental breakdown (which is what I used to think). That I just need to reduce the demands on myself and regulate myself, which I am learning how to do now and it's been life changing!

It's why I struggle to process trauma and always have done. It's why I was always so "flighty" even as a kid. Why when I'm in extreme stress I can go non-verbal. It's why I feel such deep empathy, my moral compass and need to fight social injustice is all very Autistic.

Just to add more to it, I also have ADHD, although not officially diagnosed yet as it can take up to 2 years through the NHS, I have been through the initial screening and referred by my GP. Another reason why I was missed until now is because my autism and ADHD although have similar traits also contradicted each other. The comorbidity of having both autism & adhd is between 50-70%.

It's why I need structure and can hyper focus on planning and research and love a spread sheet (autism) but at the same time struggle with the little tasks like tidying and meal planning (autism & ADHD). It's why I love being social but also get a drained social battery and have to recharge after big or prolonged social gatherings.

The combination of the autism and adhd are the reason I was so vulnerable growing up but also put myself in those worrying and dangerous situations because I had no control over my impulses. ADHD and ADD come under the same umbrella as ADHD now and it is actually a dopamine deficiency. I believe when my assessment is complete I will be diagnosed as both the inattentive and hyperactive combined. Which basically means I can be hyper (impulsive) with certain things but also a classic "daydreamer" with difficulty focussing, easily distracted and disorganised, losing things. (There's more to it, but that's in a nutshell!)

Being autistic makes a lot of things difficult for me when it comes to sensory processing. It's why I need earplugs and eye masks to even get the minimum of sleep. It's why I get stressed in certain environments because of the noise, smells and lighting. It's why I struggle to hold a conversation in a busy room if there are too many sounds at once because my autistic brain is trying to process all the sounds. My need for control of certain situations isn't because I'm being difficult it's because I'm Autistic and need boundaries and accommodations.It's why I find communicating about things like this much easier in written word.

Autism has had a bad rep back in the day but I don't take my diagnosis as a bad thing. It's let me finally understand myself and my brain for the first time in my life. It is a part of who I am and I think I'm a pretty decent human being (as is Erin!). There are so many good things being Autistic brings me. I just need a little more support and understanding with certain things. I am learning to unmask at the moment and part of that is actually telling you about it. I would love to be able to talk openly with you on it and happy to answer any questions. I just needed to write this so that I could get out all the words without having a brain freeze!

I just want to repeat, this is a good thing. I am learning and growing and finding a peace I've never had before. It's also eye-opening being able to understand so much more about myself and is brilliant for me and Erin. It's enabled me to really understand her too, we are so alike in our traits which doesn't always happen as autism is a spectrum of different things.

If you want to understand a little more about it, The Autistic Girls Network has this really useful white paper: https://autisticgirlsnetwork.org/wp-content/uploads/2022/03/Keeping-it-all-inside.pdf

Anyway that's enough of a brain dump for now. I really wanted to tell you whilst you were here but like I said I struggle to verbally vocalise things (also very Autistic trait!) and was awake at 4.30am when my brain decided to write this letter instead!! We don't have to talk about it before you leave, as I know you wanted to get off early this morning and you might want time to digest this information yourselves. I just didn't want to not tell you any longer.

Love you both
Hannah xx

I hit send on this email to them both at around 7am, knowing full well my Dad would definitely pick it up as part of his emails and news ritual in the morning even if my Mum didn't see it right away. We all busied ourselves with morning showers, breakfast and me getting our youngest off to school.

After I walked her into class, I got into my car and froze. I felt like I'd just pulled the pin of a grenade and ran away before I could see any of the damage it could cause.

FIRE IN THE HOLE!

I walked through my front door holding my breath, they were sat on the sofas, Mum crocheting, Dad probably checking the interest rate on his phone. I still wasn't quite ready for the consequences of my actions and scurried off to the kitchen where I began to load the breakfast things into the dishwasher.

Just a few minutes in to my procrastination tidying I turned to see Mum and Dad appear at the breakfast bar. Oh shit, they've definitely read it, this is it, and this is *that* conversation.

Deep breath. Exhale.

To say I wasn't prepared for happened next would be an understatement. I don't why I had built it up so much in my head (yes I do and it's called Rejection Sensitive Dysphoria). We talked for a solid hour and I know this was only possible because I had managed to write down the crucial parts first of what I wanted them to know.

I felt not only seen but also understood and that if they didn't understand something they were prepared to listen to better understand. My mum said they had always known there was something. In fact they had taken me aged 12 to see our family doctor who after speaking with me alone concluded that yes there was something but he didn't want to refer me to a psychiatrist because it would have hindered my future jobs and opportunities (it was the early 1990s). It did mean that Dad agreed to me changing schools as the doctor had said all my anxieties were school based.

I'm not going to divulge the entire conversation but that tidbit blew my mind. I was so flipping validated though, not just that but waves of relief began to rumble through me. Once my parents had left for their journey home I began to violently shake and shiver uncontrollably. My body was letting go of this particular pent up trauma that it had been carrying for so long. Armed with the therapy and knowledge I've been growing from this last 6 months, I listened to my body and just got in a warm bath to soothe myself. I removed all my demands for that day and napped too. Ooof what a day.

For Mum & Dad

As I type these words
I feel a cocktail of emotions
from relief to joy, pride to guilt

You see I never imagined
the understanding you would have
I was deluded by fear
paralysed by self preservation

Thank you for comprehending
the struggles I encountered
and the colossal undertaking
it was to build up the courage
to open up to you

I had run through umpteen
scenarios of the conversation
we would have and my jaded brain
never once conjured the reaction
that you actually had

Forgive me for not giving you
the credit you did totally deserve
for this brain of mine has been
damaged by trauma fearing the worst

Thank you for being open
to learning and understanding
for opening up your hearts
and feelings too

Four

Four pillows on my bed
as I lay down my weary head
my four limbs that ache
four sips of a water bottle
and one dry mouth
four arms entwined
in a sleep embrace
it's four am
as again I wake
the fourth time in the night
as I roll over
four lungs, gentle breaths
in the dark, still room
as my mind starts to wander
it will be time to get up soon

Oh you're still here

Each time I let you go
each tick off my journey
to find peace

I think this is it
we are done
but here you are

My mind is here
she is still teasing me
with words and memories

It seems that
despite each success
of growing

There is still
so much to know and
no actual solution

Because my dear
this brain is yours
and you have it for life

You've been Autistic
all this time
and you'll be Autistic
forever

Life is like a winter walk

Cautiously leaving the comfort of home
footsteps of trepidation across the icy ground
the wondrous sky a blanket of blue
shaded areas of snow pure white
sparkling frost decorating each leaf and twig
crunchy mud beneath your feet
boots slicing through the frozen puddles
damp breath as it dances out from your lungs
with each step there is danger but there is also beauty

Settle down now

A bedtime ritual
earplugs in place
a little read
try and quiet the mind
as you lay and ponder
all you need to do
a poem may even come to you
the calls you need to
make tomorrow
the challenges that
bring you sorrow
you read that page again
as it didn't go in
your lips feel dry
as you reach for the balm
reading again willing some calm
you're getting into it now
you feel a crumb
or an nagging itch
you adjust the bed sheet
and the folds aren't right
as you rearrange the pillow
you spy the wardrobe door ajar
and have to get up to close
whilst you're up you need a wee
back in bed you read
just another page or three
you feel the hairs move on your head
and wriggle to try and be fit for slumber
eye mask lowered time for bed
lamp turned out
how is he already
a-fucking-sleep you wonder

Floordrobe

Worn you one day robe
tried you on but didn't like it robe
couldn't decide if it was a dopamine-dress day robe
or a muted colours cos I'm over-stimulated robe
found the function to wash and dry
but not put away robes
Autism wanted to sort the robes
ADHD got bored robe
went to bed forgot you were all spread there
so lobbed you on the floordrobe

A walk on the beach

Listened to the sea
smashed some rocks
watched the sky
got wet socks

Overstimulated goblin

Being aware of my social battery
and how low it is after an event
is all well and good
when I listen to my needs
reduce demands
headphones & cosy clothes
shuffling from room to room
with my water bottle and a book
and specific playlist penetrating
my ear drums and brain
like an overstimulated goblin
retreating to my solitary place
but I wish I could manage
just for once
without the guilt

A body full of trauma

I read somewhere that we hold our trauma in our bodies. It might go someway to explain the rickety, rattly and often uselessly broken -ness that my body has felt for as long as I can remember. I have berated myself as I've gotten older and blamed a lot of it on being over-weight or for not looking after said body. However she has been broken long before I could actually blame aforementioned guilt-sticks, you know the ones we like to beat ourselves with.

Bullying was a common occurrence for my youth and I didn't realise the impact it's had on me into adulthood. In part due to the new bad-ass persona I had activated around the age of 14. Before then, I put a lot of it down to being an easy target because (wait for it) I was small, when hindsight has gifted me the real reason and that's because I was weird. Weird but also reactive which is always a joy for a bully. It wasn't just the taunts of "bible basher" in the playground either (joys of growing up to Christian parents). I was used and abused from such a young age, made a fool of in the name of entertainment and that entertainment dear readers was for the 1990's versions of mini Andrew Tates.

At age 11 or 12 years old I remember the trauma of being hauled out of the girls toilets and dragged up onto the stage of the school's Valentines Disco. I saw the activity unfolding in what felt like slow-mo before my eyes as they got boys and girls on stage so the boys could do a mock-proposal to the girls. There was a boy that I didn't even know, as he came from a different primary school to me, who had spent weeks sending his mates to ask me out on his behalf, to which I always responded "I don't know who he is".

Said boy was on the stage so I knew it wouldn't be long before my name was called to go up. Ding-a-ling - flight response engaged, I ran to the toilets. Totally in vain because I was physically removed by what felt like an angry mob and pushed up onto the stage. When the microphone was shoved in my face for a response to this weird fucking proposal performance, I said no and ran again, leaving laughter and shame in my wake.

Despite this car-crash scene of a "fun" Valentines themed night, this boy still pursued me and eventually I was worn down and agreed to being his girlfriend. We held hands and kissed like guppies, absolutely no tongues, I was a child! It did feel kind of special and I felt a bit protected now I had a new status of being someone's girlfriend (the sought after symbol of all my peers). Little did I know that it opened a new can of worms of being bullied by his much older brother. Badminton clubs, youth clubs or discos, I would go along with my new beau and if his brother was there I was physically and emotionally abused by him, who was practically a grown up in my eyes. I distinctly remember him dragging me along the sports hall floor by my ankles once because I turned up in white leggings and a spotty white t-shirt (my dress sense has always been a bit of a swerve from the norm) and he thought it would be hilarious to use me as a dust mop. Needless to say, even though my hand-holding companion was the utmost gentleman (and even once gave me the code to his bike lock - true love), the "relationship" did not last and I was feeling like an outcast loner once more.

Given that I had to be dead or dying to get a day off school, I often resorted to the tactic of pretending to be ill once at school. Traipsing myself to the school office with a "tummy ache and headache" only for my mum to always respond to their phone call with "send her back to class and see if she still feels bad in an hour" sort of thing. Putting up with school was becoming a real drag on my soul and life but I still desperately wanted to fit in. One day there was rumour of an after school fight and it was all anyone could talk about. Anyone who was *anyone* would be going along to watch the fight. I put on my favourite black platform boots (don't judge, I needed the height to see over the crowds) and walked down to see what all the fuss was about. I'd managed to get myself quite a prime viewing position at the front of the crowd, which was a good job really given that my platforms were not enough inch-wise to get me the lofty heady height I was expecting (short girl problems). It was all a huge anti-climax as one of the supposedly sparring girls hadn't turned up. The crowd became an impatient angry mob and my spidey-senses started to tingle, something shit was going to happen soon. Shouts from the crowd began to suggest someone else fight the waiting opponent and a chorus of "fight, fight, fight" ensued. Before I knew it someone had thrust me unsuspectedly into the ring. Think rabbit in headlights, that was me, how the fuck did I end up here, the smallest weirdest and most definitely the weakest person in the crowd. It's ok, my survival mode is always on high alert (thanks trauma) and off I shot. I had never run that fast in my life, and not forgetting I was also in platforms. There was a moment of debate in my mind, should I remove the footwear, but my calculations decided that would slow me down and I would be caught barefoot and vulnerable for a beating. I just kept running and I did not stop until I reached my house, panting and crying as I relayed what had happened to my parents.

My poor parents haven't actually been privy to all my perilous incidents, as unless it was unavoidable I kept it all to myself. This just meant it built up in my trauma box. I was a late bloomer and quite immature to be honest. I now know that a lot of my cluelessness in those earlier adolescent days was due to me not understanding the unwritten etiquette and not being able to read between the lines. Imagine my shock and horror when one day aged 13, hanging out with a group of kids (probably playing Nintendo) being pinned to the bed by a boy in my year, face down, in a room full of friends whilst his body trapped me there and his hands groped at my barely there breasts. I had a mouth full of duvet, no way of defending myself and literally no-one coming to my rescue. No-one ever said anything, not when it happened nor after and I was so traumatised. I remember thinking this is just what happens in life, it's what boys do, they can't help it.

Trouble seemed to follow me wherever I went. Yes I know it was me, I was the trouble. I so desperately wanted to be liked and after changing schools I fell in with some less favourable friends and my parents say this is when it all just spiralled. My injustice warrior gremlin still had me arguing back to teachers but now with added attitude. I felt like my parents hated me and by 15 years old, I moved out and in with my friend. Her mum had moved out and left my friend and her sister with their dad. A dad, that was crest fallen and in no fit state to parent two daughters and a cling-on. We pretty much did what we wanted. Living in that environment it quickly became apparent to me that this is not as fun as it initially seemed. When no-one is actually caring for you it sucks. My 16th birthday I was lonely and isolated. I went to the pub and that's where I met a slightly older boy. We ended up getting it together in my friends conservatory, which was my make-shift bedroom at their house at the time. I was purely in it for the validation but somehow ended up his girlfriend (although I never actually remember being asked!). I moved back home with my parents and would spend half my time at my new boyfriend's house.

There is so much that happened over the coming years to add to my trauma box that this chapter could end up a book in itself. I'm going to try and summarise the key moments of *what the actual fuck* so we can wrap this up. There's a real common denominator here and that is men/man-boys. I have been sexually harassed at work more times than I can count. I've been stalked by two different ex-boyfriends. Physically and emotionally abused by one particularly narcissistic specimen. Raped by a supposed friend and another time by a previously mentioned stalker ex-boyfriend. The years and years of self blame, shame and torture that followed made me feel like a useless piece of shit. Why did these things always happen to me? How did I always seem to find myself in these precarious situations and why did I attract such arseholes?

BECAUSE I WAS VULNERABLE.

It was never my fault. My need for validation made me naive, gullible and trusting. My internalisation of struggles in turn made it really hard for me to speak out and stop what was happening. I was too ashamed to tell my family that I had once again fucked up and that my boyfriend wasn't the charming, loving person he made out to be. What I found the most confusing is that I believed my own "strong girl" mask. I truly thought I was tough and how could I have let this happen to me.

Research has concluded that Autistic girls and women are 3 times more likely to be sexually assaulted than that of their Neurotypical peers. I haven't quoted a source but a quick search online throws up many stats on this, 90% of us in fact and 50% experience it before the age of 15 years old.

My body is heavy and I don't mean in kilos. My shoulders are weighted down by all of this and that's not even mentioning non-sexual traumas such as deaths, friendship breakdowns, toxic jobs and self sabotage. Rock upon figurative rock has been placed on me and it is a leaden burden I've carried with me for so many years, all without knowing my true identity. I'm Autistic, I am vulnerable and none of it was my fault.

Two worlds collide

As I unmask
and show my true
Autistic self
my trauma unravels
and unmasks too
raw and open
vulnerable and broken
a new courage evolves
as the masked
and the unmasked
become one

A kids bike

You made me laugh
being around you felt easy
when I was with you
I felt like I could
finally be me

You are so patient
and I am not
you loved me
even when I could not
love myself

We grew together
we pulled each other up
and pushed each
other higher
we were our
cheerleaders

You were the stabilisers
to my wobbly kids bike
as we ride on this
adventure together
our adventure of life

This poem is inspired not just by my husband but also my awesome friend Justine who once described him as the stabilisers to me; the chaotic child's bike.

The tank is empty

Some days the tank is simply empty
there is nothing left to give
all I have is all used up
what remains is just enough to live

Vermicelli noodles

Executive function has departed my body
my brain capacity has been fully exasperated
I know what I should and need to be doing
but the function is truly impossible
I am weak and feeble, completely exhausted
can barely string a sentence together
let alone make a decision or hold conversation
food is fuel, if I could just make some
shuffling to the kitchen and realising
I am incapable of the above stated decision
I huff and sigh and wander back forlorn
to the comfort of the fire and my blanket
replace the headphones upon my head
given up on the expectation of activity
back in my own little world of disassociation
you are there now and without a word
have recognised my needs through intuition
hand me a dish of vermicelli noodles
stir fried vegetables with just enough spice
a pot of tenderness, love and care
an unspoken love language bowl of nutrition

Inner-child healing on wheels

As I glide along
my brain stops
there is nothing but joy
the constant internal monologue paused

I can roll slowly and gracefully
instinctively slicing across the floor
sweeps and circles
a dance of happiness

The thrill of speed
as my heart races
and the breeze I create
with my own body
washes away worries

No thoughts to entertain
just pure elation
coasting a figure of eight
indulging my inner child
on roller skates

Repeat after me

I am not lazy
I am not useless
I am not hysterical
I am not a burden
I am not unlovable

I am worthy of rest
I am creative
I have valid feelings
I have many values
I am worthy of love

My deficits do not define me

I am worthy
I am worthy
I am worthy

Weirdo magnet

I use the word weirdo as a term of endearment, reclaiming and owning the fact I was always considered a bit weird. If you're feeling lost and lonely, know this, there are people out there that will love you for you. Finding them can be a little tricky at times especially when we try so hard to fit in.

Community is important and even just finding one friend amongst the sea of normies can enrich your life. Sometimes they pop up when you least expect it, it's organic and a lovely surprise. There are so many online spaces where you can meet other Neurodivergent people too. Please know that you are not alone, there are flipping millions of us. I guess that's why I felt the need to write this book. I've kept so much of me hidden away and now I'm letting her lose into the wild, expecting, hoping that my story resonates with others too because even when I've been surrounded by loved ones there's always been a lost part of me feeling like I am the only one.

Did we take over the world?

No brain, not quite.

When I set out on the intense rabbit hole of self-publishing a book, I was merely in it for the cathartic role the writing played in my post Autism diagnosis processing. Not to mention the healing properties of immersing myself into a new found hyper-focus.

My mind was blown when the book started selling beyond my friends and family. Reaching as far as Canada and the US, Australia and across Europe. The words of my readers are the very best thing in the world. It has been overwhelmingly heart warming how many humans have related to my thoughts and taken comfort from my poems. I wanted to do more and encouraged by my reader reviews, I set myself the challenge this year to get my book into a real life, physical store.

For anyone else that may have hyper-focused on self-publishing, you'll know that it does have it's restrictions and limitations (especially with the initial route that I took). So if you picked me up in a shop (or anywhere that is not from a certain worldwide conglomerate) thank you and woohoo! Ultimately, the best way I was going to achieve this was to revise the original, adding in a little sweetener for the revision, and here we are...

throws biscuits at audience

Love language

Now you've all been
able to crawl inside my brain
I feel exposed and naked
maybe you'll think I am insane

I avoid your calls
and stall our interaction
the fear is deep
too raw to face rejection

You digested every single word
page upon page of vulnerability
you know what makes me tick
the secrets of this disability

To my surprise you didn't wince
not one single falter
for now you understand the world
through the mind of your youngest daughter

You begin to send me love
in the shape of poems and memes
an authentic connection of words
all brains and feelings themed

Purple buttons

You are seven
my wish is for you to understand
your neurodivergent brain
more than we ever knew ours
and it's happening
we sit and craft
as you lift a pot of buttons
purple buttons, big and small
shaking them you said
"this is like the thoughts
inside my brain
hundreds all jumbled
it's so very busy in my head"

Hello brain

On the subject of brains, there's been a huge shift over the last twelve months in getting to know mine even more. Following my Autism diagnosis in July 2022, I was finally assessed and diagnosed with ADHD in June 2023. Not only that, I've started medication too, through the NHS Right To Choose route which although it took around a year was much swifter then if I had have waited for the standard GP referral.

It wasn't plain sailing and it infuriates me so much how inaccessible assessments are for the very people that need them. I've ranted about this enough times so will stop there for now.

Whether it's the medication or just crawling out of another burnout, I do have a new focus and motivation that I haven't seen in a long time. My judgment and decision making had been clouded for quite some time, if not forever. Absorbing book after book on any and all the information around Autism and ADHD is one hundred percent my special interest and I don't see it slowing down any time soon. (I've added more into the resources section at the end of this book). It has taught me to understand not only why my brain functions the way it does but also to work through some childhood traumas and move forward.

Rejection Sensitivity Dysphoria is hands down the most crippling part of my brain and I've been working on accepting the emotions, feeling them and then letting them go. It sounds so easy when you write it down but it really isn't. Being able to allow myself to have the feelings and not spiral over them has not happened over night and I don't even know if this will last but hey, this is an update and it's where we are now, my brain and I.

Earlier in this book, I shared my letter to my parents telling them about my diagnosis and their reaction. Well imagine how much my stomach dropped out of my arse when my Mum posted on Facebook "we've ordered a copy" after I had plucked up the courage to fully out myself publicly on my personal social media. Who's silly idea was it to put all my inner most feelings into paperback for all to read? I nigh on triggered a panic attack or meltdown, whatever it was. My temperature shot up, I was sweating, couldn't breath and felt so sick. Regret, the regret was strong.

As a steadfast bottler-upper, a worrier of being a burden on literally anyone for having feelings or any minor inconvenience throwing me head first into people pleasing mode. This was a mistake. What have I done. People I knew were buying it and reading it in a day. After the initial complete existential dismay, I had a little word with myself and my brain. Feedback was coming in and it was good, better than good. Wow, ok, this isn't so bad.

It was time to call my parents back after not daring to answer the phone to them post book purchase. Apparently dad read it first and mum was halfway through. Dad was very complimentary (despite the swears) and my mum said she feels like she understands me better. At forty years old, I wrote a book and my mum read it and understood. I'm not suggesting that the only way to connect with your parents is by penning a memoir but bloody Nora I didn't think the response was going to be so positive, so warm and validating.

There isn't a family get together now where we don't talk about Autism or ADHD. Mum recognising many Autistic traits in herself. Not long after this my mum, (the woman who rarely buys random things *just because*) handed me a little something she saw in a gift shop, because (and I quote) "I saw it and thought of you". She immediately begins to downplay it, it was only a couple of quid, it's nothing special. I open the bag and inside is an A5 sized zipped purse, embossed on the front are the words:

HANNAH
TAKE ME AS I AM
OR WATCH ME
AS I GO

Speechless, I tell you! I couldn't really find the words to how much this little "couple of quid" purse meant to me. Firstly, the fact that someone had thought of me when I was not in sight. Secondly, because I love the message, the love language of understanding boundaries all tied up in one little stamped quote.

Sugar-coated VA

There's a tiny little
virtual assistant
inside this sugar coat
a pill designed to
organise the thoughts
to focus the attention
channel that creativity
there was no miracle quiet
no stillness that made me weep

The filing system
that was once a mess
now neatly packed
somehow prioritised
inside my mind there are still
umpteen-thousand things
yet a lower level of stress
the ideas continue
to abundantly flow
no more chronic overwhelm
and above all, at last I fucking sleep

There is still a floordrobe in my bedroom, apparently medication can help focus your mind, alas it cannot force that focus on the tasks that are not that interesting nor that important to your Neurodivergent brain.

Not a genie

Years of masking
trying to figure out who I am
using booze to bring out
the palatable Hannah
character in a can

Unmasking is an adventure
something new at every turn
my personality isn't inside a bottle
is the latest thing I've learnt

I have just completed my first totally sober Christmas
takes bow

Representation

The year I learnt about my brain
the world learnt some more too
as we watched in awe
films of each sharing their stories
the understanding grew

It felt like all were listening
as I sat on my sofa sobbing
the words portrayed
and masking explained
my vulnerability reflecting
in people on the screen

Not knowing who I was
for years - my life
an alien in disguise
to see the people just like me
a warm and welcome surprise

Holy Sh**. Get out of my brain

The sweet-nothings that landed in my WhatsApp from Flo as we chatted about my poems.

Let's do a quick rewind. In the midst of my Autism awakening, multiple existential crises, burnout, chronic overwhelm, exhaustion and a mind swarming of things I needed to do as well as all the seemingly simple tasks I couldn't physically even start. I sat watching a documentary and I began to weep.

The impulse hit to share on my (relatively new) TikTok account, my raw emotions of how the show *Inside Our Autistic Minds* made me feel. Not thinking much more of it, I clicked post. Well it popped off (is that what the kids say?). Suddenly there were all these people sharing in my emotions and relating to me, how the representation made them feel too. I think it actually finally gave me the courage to go live with my book. There are people out there that want to be heard, that want to know they're not alone and I'd written so much from my soul that I could do just that.

With my new found confidence I shared about the program on my personal Facebook profile:
"If you are Autistic or know someone that is, then watch this, it's incredible, second episode is next week".
A cheeky little precursor to posting about my very personal book.

To my surprise a good friend of mine tells me she needs to watch it because her friend Flo is on the program. At this point I couldn't believe how small the world really is because I thought Flo was a legend. Finally seeing an Autistic woman on national television was just incredible. Little miss bravado pants over here decided to ask my friend to introduce us. The connection I felt with Flo was so strong, especially as her film was a letter to her mum, just like I had written to mine. I wanted to give Flo a copy of my book. We began to message each other. Her sister-in-law had just sent her my TikTok post (again frighteningly small world) and we quickly discovered we lived just thirty minutes away and so the hand delivery of Mess is Progress was arranged.

Nerves and anxiety rippled through my body before meeting Flo (new people anxiety) but as soon as we sat down and began to chat it was a breath of fresh air. Autism is a spectrum but crikey did we have a lot in common. Even down to our special interests; genealogy being one and the unofficial Autism uniform of our Lucy & Yak dungarees.

After I left and in the following days I got blow by blow reactions pinging up on WhatsApp from Flo that truly meant the absolute world to me. What I wasn't quite prepared for was the poem that she wrote back to me when she finished.

At this point I was drowning in a pool of my own tears.

Representation matters.

Epilogue

Being open about my diagnoses has not only set me free, but it has given my children time and space to understand themselves too. Our entire family are on this learning curve of discovery, together. Listening to my youngest express her emotions and how it feels inside her brain makes my heart ache a little. Not in a bad way, in a healing way. Knowing that she has a deeper knowledge of who she is at such a young age, brings me so much hope. It's what cycle-breaking is all about, is it not? It may have been woefully late for myself and my older kids to have grasped our grey-matter's nuances but we are getting there. This process has enabled us to give the gift of recognition and identity to a child, if born a decade ago would have completely flown under the radar.

Just a few weeks ago, in the library she asked if she could take out a book about ADHD, of which I obliged. We found one aimed at her age and after reading about half of it she declared it was rubbish because it didn't teach her anything she didn't already know. She wasn't being contrary, she was right. We've armed her with the information through casually talking, honestly, openly and authentically about being Neurodivergent.

Knowledge is power. It's not just reading the dictionary and thesaurus as a child - the Autistic coping mechanism to feeling different or because we felt stupid due to our un-diagnosed ADHD (we all did it, didn't we?). This special interest of mine makes me feel stronger as a human being. Healthier even.

It's full on empowerment.

Acknowledgements

Zena my wonderful therapist, thank you for your raw and honest reactions to my poetry and for encouraging me that "these need to be heard".

Amy, a wonderful random stranger I "met" on TikTok. A fellow AuDHDer, who took the time to not only go through my manuscript to help me fine-tune it, but also gave me feedback on the content that truly warmed my soul.

Flo - for the beautiful poem review that is now pride of place as the Foreword in this book. Thank you. And thank you for doing the documentary, your openness and authenticity has reached so many people.

During my post diagnosis burnout and therapy sessions, we were also going through an extension project on our home. Our builder gave me regular pep talks through the destruction phases of "Mess is progress" and never has a random saying resonated with me so deeply on a personal level.

Huge thank you to my Autistic and ADHD friends in the photography community. Not only have you helped me work through some shit you've also warmed my soul with your wisdom, support and unwavering positivity for me to try something I've never done before. Having your points of view in the early stages has been priceless. You are incredible women.

To Sara, Jamie, Vanina, Tash and Emily, my weirdo magnet mates. Thank you for entertaining the copious amounts of Autism chat, having my special interest heard is a gift. I value you all and your friendship means so much to me.

Pickle, I still can't believe to this day that you thought I was brilliant. You were the first person to openly voice that I genuinely meant something to them and it blew my mind. To Justine, Rachel, Adam, Emily and Jocelyn, my treasure box friends from all the eras. You mean so much to me even when I'm rubbish at getting in touch.

My sister Gemma for all the hours and hours we've spent talking about Autism and ADHD and also just because I love you. Sharing DNA with my best friend is pretty special, thank you.

Thank you Erin for being you. You inspire me and motivated me to actually go through with this book, cheerleading and listening to my ideas. Relating to my words and affirming to me the content I was so feverishly constructing had value. To my oldest manchild Jake, you make me so proud and my youngest Mila who is still teaching me so much about being a parent all these years later. Nicola, Claire, Mum & Dad - I know my boundaries may have confused you all at times but thank you for not giving up on me, I love you.

The biggest thank you has been reserved for my ever-patient husband. We have all been through a huge learning curve of adaption. Understanding (finally) what it means to be a Neurodivergent household.

Burnout is such a tough place to be but knowing that you've got my back throughout has made it all that much easier. Also the late night scribblings in my notebook and PJ days typing up words instead of giving you attention when I probably should have been! The big gestures of basically doing all the daily chores on my bad days and the little gestures of finding me a new fidget toy without me even asking. Your comprehension of my determination when I told you I was going to write a book and unwavering support always. You know I love a challenge or a project but are also fully aware of how much I will hyper-focus on it until it's done whilst everything else falls by the wayside. Thanks for being you and making me laugh when I truly need to.

Glossary of terms (Hannah's way)

I know it's not tradition to write about what a glossary entails but hey I'm non-traditional human being. I wanted to put these words into the book for a reference, so that readers could go back to them when necessary. One of the practical bits of advice I can give you if you think you're Autistic or have just been diagnosed, is to familiarise yourself with as many of these terms as possible. We've grown up with bucket loads of shitty labels, shame and confusion. Understanding what it is to be Autistic and/or ADHD will help you shed those labels piece by piece. You become more accepting and forgiving to yourself when you have the right words. Having the correct vocabulary can also help you express to friends and family what life is like for you and why diagnosis and understanding is important. I hope it helps you heal as it does for me.

Autistic/Autism - Being an Autistic person means that you have a neurological brain condition where your brain works differently. This can lead to difficulty with a spectrum of things from social communication and processing based on a Neurotypical world. I use identity first language throughout the book because I am Autistic and always will be, I don't *have* Autism, it's not something I can put down or get rid of. Likewise I don't say I have ASD.

Ableism - Internalised or otherwise. There's no escaping the fact we live in an ableist society. It is not made for disabled people and Autism is a disability.

You can be disabled and still be ableist at the same time. It is to discriminate a person due to their disability. This includes both physical and invisible disabilities. Such as not providing physical access to a property for someone in a wheelchair, to not providing accommodations to an Autistic person to meet their needs. I am still working on my own internalised ableism (which is mostly directed at myself).

Burnout - Quite the hot phrase and not surprising in the current climate and state of the world. However Autistic burnout has a different twist to it, it's not just brought on by a crashing economy, under-funded schools and a cost of living crisis. When an Autistic person hits burnout, it can be contributed by the above factors however the overwhelm and over-stimulation is a huge part. We are physically assaulted by sensory input, lights, smells, sounds and yes social injustice. Our bodies and brains shutdown and we cannot do anything. Emotionally we are all over the place and even the simplest of things are impossible.

Comorbidity - The presence of not one but two (or more) conditions in the same person. For example Autistic women are statistically (50-70%) more likely to be both Autistic and ADHD, more likely to have bowel problems, auto-immune conditions and so on.

Deficits - The dictionary definition is *"the amount by which something, especially a sum of money, is too small."* In the world of autism, it's basically countless lists of what you cannot do. Sadly the entire DSM-5 is made up of what you cannot do compared to your Neurotypical peers.

DSM-5 - The Diagnostic and Statistical Manual of Mental Disorders. It's the what Autism and ADHD assessments are based on, the "5" is just the number correlating to the latest edition. When you are assessed you have to meet the criteria in the different sections such as; social-emotional, communicative behaviours and social interactions, deficits in developing, maintaining and understanding relationships, routine/rigid thinking, special interests and hyper-reactivity to sensory input. I forget the full list and there is a certain number of ticks for each section to result in a diagnosis but you get the gist.

Dopamine - It's the good shit - a hormone that makes you feel a high and ND people can be seriously lacking in it. It can cause impulse spending and financial issues. It messes with all the regulation that we actually need. When we are really lacking it makes executive function nigh on impossible. It can also make us have a really poor diet as we try and eat our way to Dopamine.

Dysregulation - Emotional dysregulation, when I cannot control my feelings. I might have slumped and sometimes even confused bodily signals with sadness. It affects my nervous system and I have to do specific things to regulate again. It can be something small like a stim toy or it may need a more drastic tactic such as getting in the sea. If I don't work on regulating then I will hit a meltdown.

Echolalia - Repeating words, sounds or phrases. Think Buddy the Elf when he hears the name "Francisco" and repeats it because he really likes how the sound comes from his mouth. It can be repeated in the moment, saved for later or on loop in your head for the foreseeable.

Executive Function/Dysfunction - I personally prefer to say that my executive function is low because I'm just sick of the sight of Dys-anything. It's a symptom that blocks my ability to manage the menial tasks of self care or day to day jobs. From showering to putting clean pants on, meal planning and general household chores. It causes struggles with long term goals, time blindness and organisation. It affects my emotions and my impulsivity.

Interoception - It's another sense to add to touch, sight, feel, taste, sound. Interoception is the messages from inside the body which can be impacted as an Autistic person. You can be hypersensitive to them or be completely the opposite way and not feel them at all. Such as feelings internally with your organs, eg heart beats, need to pee, hunger, temperature, gut and so on.

Masking - A safety tool that ND people use consciously or subconsciously to fit in and suppress certain behaviours that others may find weird. This includes things such as stimming, intense interests and/or emotions. It's exhausting and damaging.

Meltdown - Not. A. Tantrum. Just had to get that off my chest first. It is the uncontrollable reaction to a situation either emotionally or sensory triggered. We usually have a lot of shame around them, because of the complete loss of control. My worst have included physically harming myself in the process, accompanied with sobbing and rocking.

Mirroring/Mimicking - Not always intentional and also a safety feature for our Autistic brains. It's part of masking and enables us to work out how we "should" be behaving in society. Our trauma makes us very conscious of expectations and we can default to copying to fit in or to be safe.

Neurodivergent - A different neurological functioning brain to what is considered normal, used for Autism, ADHD, OCD, Dyslexia and many other conditions.

RSD - Rejection Sensitivity Dysphoria - If you haven't come across this before, hopefully you have a better understanding from my book. RSD is a common issue with Neurodivergent people and it sucks. It's physical and intense pain from the fear, of rejection, actual or perceived.

Sensory Processing - The way in which your brain processes sensory input. As an Autistic person we usually (but not always) have sensory processing disorder (SPD) which means we can be adverse to certain sounds, food textures and clothing. It can also make us sensory seek - swinging, rocking, fluffy blankets all feel nice (to me anyway, all Autistics are different).

Stimming - Repetitive movements or noises that help us regulate. I vape and I wish I didn't but I know it's a stim. I fiddle with my hair constantly, scratch and rub at my skin. Dancing is a great way to stim as is singing or repeating sounds, words or phrases. I also constantly pick at the skin on my fingers and thumbs. Stimming also helps me concentrate on some tasks.

Helpful resources

Reading list
Girls and Autism: Educational, Family and Personal Perspectives - *Barry Carpenter, Francesca Happé & Jo Egerton*
Unmasking Autism - *Dr Devon Price*
Helping Autistic Teens to Manage their Anxiety - *Dr Theresa Kid*
Understanding ADHD in Girls & Women - *Joanne Steer*
Nurturing Your Autistic Young Person - *Cathy Wassell*
A Different Way to Learn - *Dr Naomi Fisher*
Drama Queen - *Sara Gibbs*
Ten Steps to Nanette - *Hannah Gadsby*
Strong Female Character - *Fern Brady*
A Kind of Spark - *Elle McNicoll*

Online resources
BBC iPlayer - *Inside Our Autistic Minds*
BBC iPlayer - Christine McGuinness, *Unmasking My Autism*
Autistic Girls Network
(Facebook page, private group and website)
https://www.nhs.uk/using-the-nhs/about-the-nhs/your-choices-in-the-nhs/
https://www.gov.uk/access-to-work
https://embrace-autism.com/

Podcasts
ADHD As Females (ADHDAF)
The Late Discovered Club
The ADHD Adults

Your reviews count

As a self-published writer your reviews mean a lot (forcibly shoves RSD out the door, slams it shut and slides the bolt across).

Our voices and stories need to be heard, the more we share, the less alone we feel. Please take a brief moment to leave a review, I will be forever grateful.

For updates on future books check out:
hannahpoems.co.uk

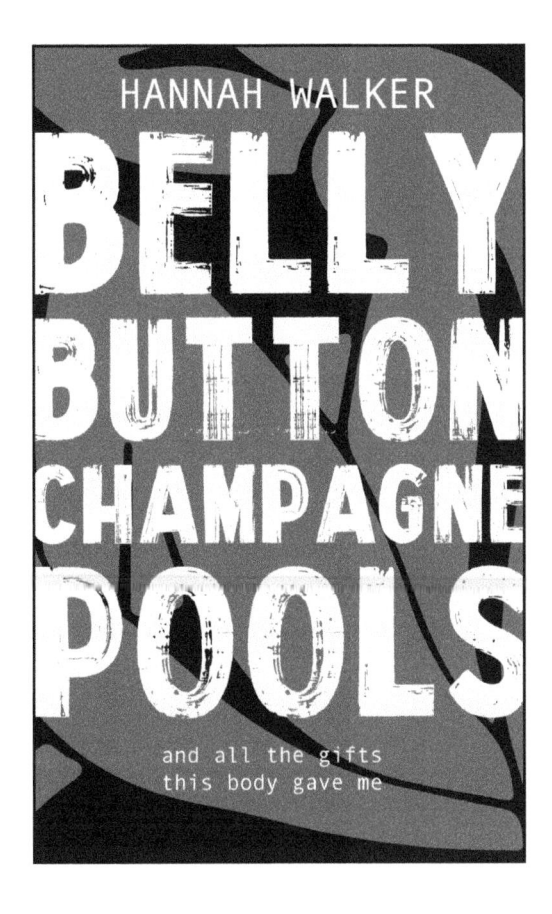

HANNAH WALKER

BELLY BUTTON CHAMPAGNE POOLS

and all the gifts this body gave me

From sex hair to hammer toes, our bodies hold the stories of crusades, calamities and connection.
Belly Button Champagne Pools unlocks the tales on an anatomy adventure, through honest and witty poetry and prose.

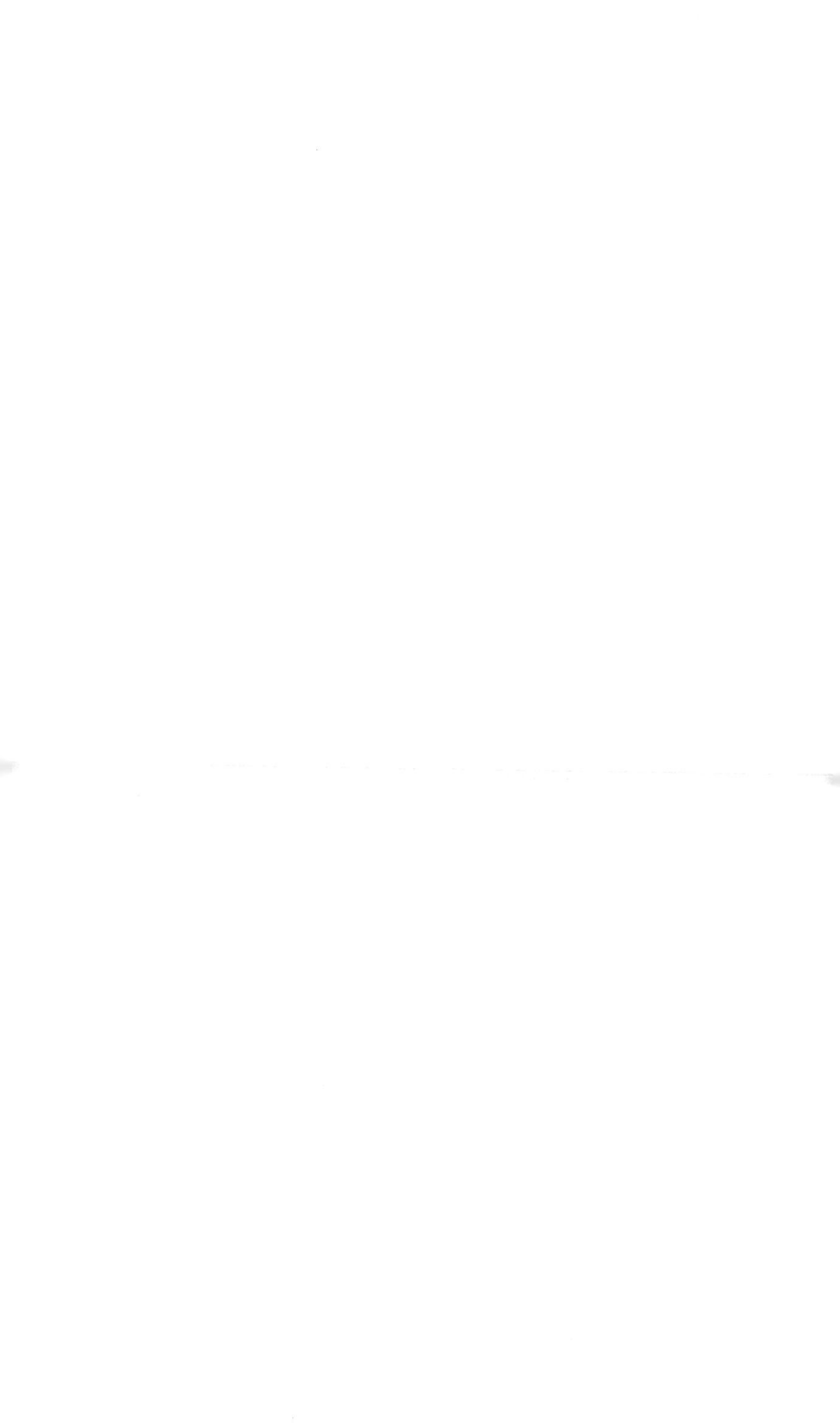

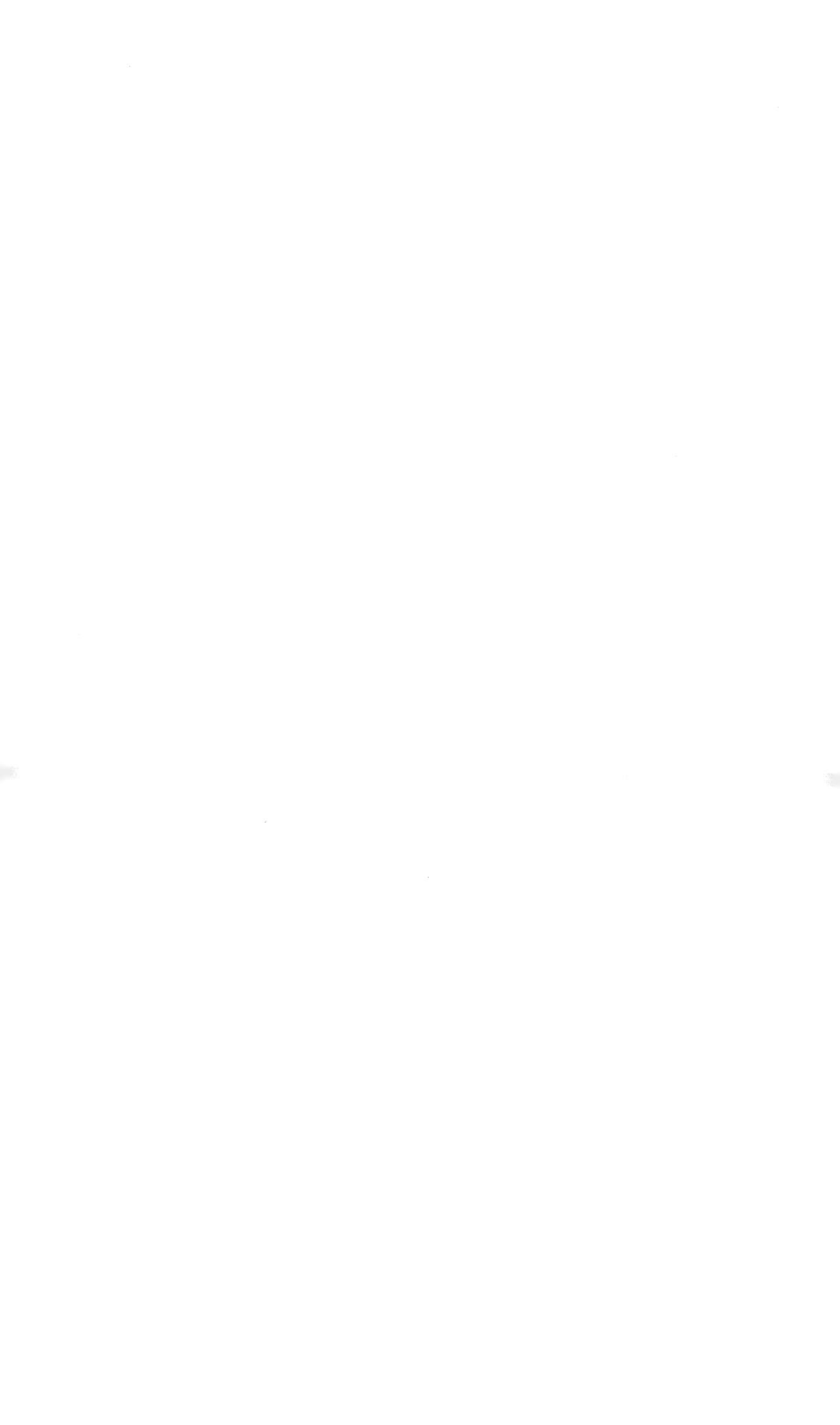

Milton Keynes UK
Ingram Content Group UK Ltd.
UKHW031025170324
439567UK00005B/59

9 781738 510306